'Fascinating and [...] [...] [...] nfides
in us the joys and agony of facial surgery.'
Dr Richard Shepherd, Consultant Forensic Pathologist
and bestselling author of *Unnatural Causes*

WITHDRAWN

'There's a vicarious thrill to being let into this insider
zone . . . inspires wonder at all that modern medicine
can achieve.'
TLS

'A wonderful book for everyone who has a zest
for the healing power of curiosity.'
Professor Gordon Turnbull, Consultant Psychiatrist
and author of *Trauma*

'Enjoyable and compelling.'
Mail on Sunday

'The pages sear the mind's eye with stories of
tragedy, loss, hope, life and death.'
Evening Times

True stories of life, death

and transformation from

my career as a facial surgeon

face to face

Professor Jim McCaul

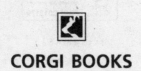

CORGI BOOKS

TRANSWORLD PUBLISHERS
61–63 Uxbridge Road, London W5 5SA
www.penguin.co.uk

Transworld is part of the Penguin Random House group of companies
whose addresses can be found at global.penguinrandomhouse.com

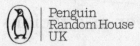

First published in Great Britain in 2018 by Bantam Press
an imprint of Transworld Publishers
Corgi edition published 2019

A CIP catalogue record for this book
is available from the British Library.

ISBN 9780552174336

Typeset in 11.04/14.9pt Minion Pro by Jouve (UK), Milton Keynes.
Printed and bound in Great Britain by Clays Ltd, Elcograf S.p.A.

Penguin Random House is committed to a sustainable future
for our business, our readers and our planet. This book is made
from Forest Stewardship Council® certified paper.

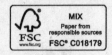

1 3 5 7 9 10 8 6 4 2

This book is dedicated to maxillofacial patients, from soldiers of the Great War to the present day and beyond. Also to maxillofacial surgeons past, present and future, some of whom I hope might one day be inspired by this book to join the speciality.

Author's Note

Throughout the book, when discussing surgical procedures, I have generally used 'we' rather than 'I', not because I think I'm a member of the Royal Family entitled to use 'the royal We', but because it emphasizes that surgery is always a team operation, involving a dozen or more people, all of whom are equally vital to the success of the procedure.

Although all the patients whose cases have been discussed here have given their permission for the details to be made public, to preserve their privacy I have changed their names and identifying details.

The individual on whom we operate is more than a physiological mechanism. He thinks, he fears, his body trembles if he lacks the comfort of a sympathetic face. For him nothing will replace the salutary contact with his surgeon, the exchange of looks, the feeling that the doctor has taken charge, with the certainty, at least apparent, of winning.

René Leriche (1879-1955),
The Philosophy of Surgery (tr. Roberta Hurwitz)

Introduction

I'VE BEEN A maxillofacial surgeon for over twenty years, carrying out surgery and microsurgery to the face and neck to repair damage from disease, accident or violence. It is hugely rewarding but intensely demanding work, performing surgery on structures some of which are almost invisible to the naked eye in the full knowledge that one slip may leave the patient permanently disfigured or even at risk of their life.

However, writing this book has been even more demanding, one of the hardest things I've ever had to do, because in order to write it I've had to lower the 'professional shield' that all surgeons must wield. My patients are individual human beings and are treated with respect and dignity at all times, but I cannot allow myself to become too closely involved in their emotional lives, personal tragedies, hopes and fears: without the professional shield I could dissolve in the overwhelming nature of the problems I and my patients face – and I would then be useless to them.

I and my team carry out what is commonly known as 'plastic surgery'. That tends to evoke images of breast implants, face-lifts, tummy tucks and the rest of the panoply of cosmetic procedures with which people – men and women – seek to remedy real or imagined defects in their looks and prolong their youthful appearance. It is perfectly legitimate for people to undergo cosmetic surgery if they wish, of course, but it is not the principal reason why I and my team operate on my patients.

1

Many benign or malignant facial conditions require surgical interventions that may affect not only a patient's looks but also their ability to speak, eat and swallow. As the name suggests (*maxilla* is Latin for 'jawbone'), a maxillofacial surgeon's task is to find a way to correct damage to the patient's facial and oral functions and appearance without compromising the treatment of their medical condition. We excise cancerous tumours and repair traumatic damage, but we also aim to restore our patients' former appearance, not to satisfy their personal vanity but to give them back their self-respect and dignity, their happiness and their lives.

All surgeons carry out procedures that enhance their patients' lives and are often life-saving, but maxillofacial surgery carries an additional burden of significance and responsibility. A livid breastbone-to-navel scar left after open heart surgery might be a little unsightly but it will usually be covered by a patient's clothes, and even when exposed on a Mediterranean holiday it is not a repugnant or frightening sight. Similarly the scar left on a woman's abdomen by a Caesarean section will be concealed by her everyday clothes or hidden by her bikini at the beach and will have no impact on people's perceptions of her. However, because our identity is so closely tied up with the face that we present to the world, facial scarring, whether it is caused by trauma or disease, or by the surgery to cure them, has an immediate and potentially profound impact on our relations with those around us.

The face is the site of four of the five human senses – sight, smell, hearing and taste – but it also performs an even more vital function because to a great extent the human sense of self is based on our perceptions of what we look like and what others see when they look at us. We are all 'hardwired' to appreciate and judge facial appearance; it is pre-programmed into the human brain and is powerfully emotive. The abhorrence of the human psyche for a disfigured or distorted human face is clear through the entire history of the horror genre.

Looking round a café or a bar, we read faces like barcodes and we know almost instinctively which are the 'attractive' and 'unattractive' faces, though the physical differences that cause those judgements to be made can be tiny. Even after twenty-five years working in my field I'm still very aware of how the smallest modification can produce a startling improvement in the overall harmony of a person's face; it still stuns me.

Think how much your identity and sense of self is vested in what you see in the bathroom mirror every morning. Now imagine the impact on you if the face you've known all your life has been so ravaged by cancer, an accident, a fall, a beating, a car crash or a gunshot wound that it is barely recognizable. When you leave the house, your disfigurement is met everywhere by looks of shock. Some friends and acquaintances cross the street to avoid you, and you must endure stares and cruel comments from strangers, adults and children alike. Even close friends and family members flinch at the sight of your face. Some find these reactions so upsetting that they become virtual recluses, never leaving their houses for fear of the reactions they'll provoke.

Now imagine how it feels when, after microsurgery, the person you remember, but had given up all hope of ever seeing again, is once more looking back at you from the mirror. Knowing my team has helped to bring about such a transformation, rebuilding not just a face but a life, is a truly wonderful feeling.

We have helped countless individuals over the years, but a patient's joy after a successful procedure – a joy which we are privileged to share – still brings a lump to every throat. It's why I became a maxillofacial surgeon in the first place and why I still feel the same excitement as I approach the operating theatre today as I did when I was a young trainee twenty-five years ago.

Jim McCaul
MARCH 2018

1

LIKE MOST SURGEONS, whatever their speciality, there is no such thing as a 'typical case' for me, because each one presents different challenges. However, about 80 per cent of my work involves treating patients with tumours of the face, mouth or neck. Most of them are major surgical cases – any procedure lasting more than three hours is defined as a major case, though we will often be operating for eight to twelve hours, and in rare cases where the blood vessels that should be draining a transplanted flap simply refuse to do so, it can take anything up to twenty-four hours. So the major cases are always the most stressful, but they are also the most fulfilling when everything goes well.

The night before carrying out a major operation is never a late night; I always want a good rest with no big stress and hassle. Monday is not a bad day to do major operations, though it does tend to mess up Sunday as a day for socializing: a gin and tonic and a wander in the garden or a glass of wine with dinner is about the limit of it. I always have fixed operating days and I'm always excited the night before a big case, so it's never a problem to get up early in the morning. I shower and shave, then make a good, strong cup of coffee with freshly ground beans – a habit I acquired when working in Miami – and set off down the stairs to the car with my coffee in one hand and a piece of toast in the other.

The stuff I need to have with me is already in a bag in the back of the car, including the wooden box containing my operating loupes (with 2.5 times magnification), the Bose speakers for my music, some snacks and a bottle of water. I also have my camera bag containing my Nikon D700 SLR. I've taken photographs of my cases ever since my mum and dad bought me a Nikon camera as a present when I graduated in Dentistry. When I was working in North America, I discovered that surgeons there also photograph absolutely every case for their individual surgical log-books as evidence that the procedure actually took place, because without the photographs as proof, it is not considered to have occurred. Given the litigious nature of American society, these images can also be drawn on as evidence if necessary.

So with the consent of my patients, I photograph every stage of every procedure. But that's not for protection against potential lawsuits if anything goes wrong, it's to allow me to train the other surgeons present by going through each stage with them afterwards. It also allows me to review the entire operation myself and analyse whether we could have improved any part of it. If anything has not gone as well as we had hoped, we work as a team in our hospital 'Morbidity and Mortality' meetings to work out where we can get better. So it's always a part of the pre-operative briefing, where we talk through the procedure, to say 'We'll take a photograph of that and one of that' – just to show, for example, that we couldn't get any more clearance around a particular area when excising a tumour, because under it is the carotid artery which supplies about half the brain with blood, so we had better leave it where it is.

With further patient permission, I also use the images as

illustrations during lectures when I teach groups of trainee surgeons. Recently, while video-linking from London for a large training event, I used them to teach more than 300 Iraqi surgeons who – first under Saddam Hussein's dictatorship and then during the chaos and near civil war that engulfed Iraq following the US-led invasion of the country – had been cut off from advances in Western medicine for almost thirty years. I am eternally grateful to all the patients who have given me permission to teach using their photos and I always acknowledge this when I'm speaking publicly.

On major surgery days, the sense of anticipation and excitement keeps building in me all the way to the hospital. When I was small I used to get very excited when I was going swimming with my dad at the pool in Johnstone near Glasgow, and I still get a bit of that kind of feeling when I'm walking in the door of the hospital to get ready for a big case. Although one or two of the hospitals where I usually work have very imposing main entrances, I and my fellow surgeons hardly ever use them: we always tend to come and go through the entrance nearest to the operating theatre, and that is invariably round the back, near the rubbish bins.

The familiar tang of antiseptic is always the first thing I notice as I walk through the hospital doors. It is 150 years since Joseph Lister first used a carboxylic acid spray in Glasgow Royal Infirmary, before treating a seven-year-old boy with a fractured kneecap. Unlike most patients at the time, the boy didn't get an infection, and Lister's use of disinfectant and other aseptic methods including hand-washing and sterilizing instruments became the accepted practice. So that smell of antiseptic is always a reminder to me that before Lister pioneered its use, having an operation was an absolute lottery, and if you were a patient, all too often you had a losing ticket, because back then, even when a procedure was completely successful, 50 per cent of patients died after surgery, most of them from post-operative infections that were so prevalent they were known simply as 'ward fever' or 'hospitalism'.

As well as the antiseptic aroma, a wave of warm air also greets me, because the ambient temperature in hospitals is set for people in their pyjamas, not those who are fully dressed. That always makes it much too hot for the medical and nursing staff, but it is something we accept and deal with because we know that hospitals are not run for our comfort, but that of the patients.

I pass through two security doors and, as always, the nearer I get to the operating theatre, the more tangible is the buzz in the atmosphere. Nurses in scrubs are always bustling around with trolleys and instruments and I say a few hellos on my way to the theatre suite.

I travel to work in 'civvies' on operating days and head straight for the changing rooms, hang my clothes in my locker and put on my theatre scrubs and hat, ready for action. My next task is to go and see my patients on the ward. They are inevitably anxious and more than a little fearful, for in many cases there may be fatal consequences if the operation is not success-ful, so I want their first sight of me on the day they have been anticipating and quite possibly dreading to be in a calm envir-onment, not the bustle of the theatre suite. I feel that it is important for them to see me looking cool, confident and ready to go before they come down to the theatre, and I try to speak to them in a calm, reassuring way, just saying, 'How are you doing? We're all set and you don't have to worry about a thing. I've a great team working with me and everything is going to be absolutely fine. I'll see you when you're back on the ward and awake again.' A few words from me are not going to wave a magic wand and make their fears completely disappear, of course, but I hope they give them some reassurance.

After seeing my patients, I walk back down to the theatre suite, and as I open the door of the operating theatre I can feel the familiar out-rush of air through the opening from the brightly lit room beyond. There is a laminar airflow in operating theatres, a system of circulating filtered air in parallel-flowing planes to reduce the risk of airborne contaminants or chemical pollutants entering the room. Pure, sterile air is constantly pumped in to keep the room at a higher pressure than the surrounding area, ensuring that any airflow is only one way – from in to out, and not out to in – so no foreign particles can get into the theatre on an air current. It does tend to make it a very dry environment, leading to severe dehydration if you're working in there for any length of time, and the major operations we do often take all day, and sometimes all night as well.

The full surgical team is normally eleven or twelve strong: an anaesthetist who has his or her own nurse; two consultants; two registrars (trainee surgeons); two 'scrubbed-in' (gloved, gowned and fully sterile) scrub nurses who handle the sterile instruments for the surgeons; and three or four other nurses who are not scrubbed-in and who act as 'gofers' bringing other instruments, swabs and anything else the scrub nurses or surgeons ask for.

Although autoclaves are still sometimes used, our instruments are usually sterilized not by heat or liquids but by sonic micro-pulses that set the instruments vibrating and 'shake off' any molecules adhering to them. Anything, such as a fresh set of swabs, brought into the theatre by the non-scrubbed-in nurses is in a double-wrapped pack. The first nurse tears the outer wrapping but does not touch the sterile second wrapping inside. She holds out the pack to the scrub nurse who takes the sterile instrument in its sterile pack without touching the outer wrapping, opens it, and passes the swab to the surgeon. When operating, surgeons tend to be quiet and almost still, but the further down the chain of command you go the more move-ment and the more noise there is, and the non-scrubbed-in nurses bustling in and out of the theatre are always the most chatty.

Before the patient is brought down from the ward to the the-atre suite, I always hold a briefing. The entire surgical team stands in a circle, wearing scrubs and theatre hats but not scrubbed-in and gowned at this stage. We all wear blue scrubs that are clean but some still bear the faint marks of stains from previous oper-ations that no amount of boil-washing and sterilizing can apparently remove. They also tend to be ill-fitting – the product, I believe, of a 'one size fits all' rule adopted by hospital adminis-trators. Almost all hospital scrubs seem to be XL size, so the bodies of the more well-built staff may be straining at the fabric of their scrubs while the more petite members can practically turn round inside theirs without removing them. Everyone wears clogs or plastic crocs on their feet and they provide some of the few flashes of strong colour in the operating theatre. A few of the team wear red crocs, and one flamboyant nurse has pink ones with stencilled flowers on them. Mine are always white, but by the end of an operation they are a different colour because surgeons' crocs are always splashed with blood and other bodily fluids that have dripped from the operating table. The hazardous waste bins in the operating theatre are bright orange and yellow but almost everything else in there is silver, white or muted tones of pale blue and pale green.

I usually open the briefing by saying something like 'Welcome to Theatre 12, which as you know on alternate Mondays [the days when I operate there] is the best one!' The joke might be getting more than a little tired by now but it is not only a way of breaking the ice and defusing the tension, it also reminds everyone that we are forever aiming to achieve the highest possible professional standards.

The briefing is a time to stress the value of the contributions of all the team members. I go around the group and we all introduce ourselves and outline our particular roles. Whenever there is a new face among the staff or trainees, or a new medical, dental or work experience student present, I make a point of introducing them myself, so that they feel a bit more involved in the procedure. I reinforce that by telling them, 'You're part of the team when you're here, you're not peripheral to it,' because often they feel their only role is to touch something sterile and get shouted at . . . which of course does happen! The key message is that this is a professional team, caring collectively for the patient on the operating table, and they should carry this culture forward throughout their medical or nursing careers. However, I'm always 'Consultant Surgeon Jim McCaul' in briefings, not because I want to stand on ceremony or hide behind my title, but because it emphasizes that, although it is a collaborative process, I am the team leader and the ultimate responsibility for decision-making rests with me.

There is often a mixture of operations on our list and we discuss them in the order they are written on the paper, even if we then change the list order at the end. Sometimes there will only be one major case on our list, which we know will take the whole day – and sometimes more than that – to complete.

The briefing needs to be done before the patient is brought down to the theatre suite and it can be a hassle to organize because everyone must be present for it. Sometimes people are preparing instrument trays, or checking vital equipment, or making sure the detailed cross-sectional imaging is available, or the registrar is on a ward round, or one of the theatre staff is not starting until ten o'clock because they're on a later shift . . . and we have to hang around until everyone has assembled. There is no question of starting without someone; they must all be in the room for the briefing, because any operation is a collaborative process. Input is welcome from anyone, and if everyone knows the plan, the chance of anything going wrong is reduced and the reaction if it does will be quicker and smoother.

I often ask questions of the team members to increase their sense of involvement, because we need an environment in which everyone is comfortable about speaking up and expressing an opinion: even though I have three decades of training and experience behind me, I still don't know everything; you never stop learning. It's a little like the 'Chinese Parliaments' that the SAS hold before their very different kinds of operations. In the SAS, everyone is free to participate in the discussion when the operation is being planned, and the one unbreakable rule is that if you do not voice your opinion during the briefing you do not get to make criticisms of how the operation was carried out afterwards. In the same way, the one thing I never want to hear when something has gone wrong with a procedure is 'I wasn't sure about that before we started'. If you weren't sure, you should have said so in the briefing before we began.

The team then talks through the various processes we'll be following during the operation and the need for certain procedures and drugs. These include antibiotics to prevent infection, administered just before we start operating; tapered compression stockings and pneumatic calf pumps on the legs to prevent clots forming in deep veins, which can then break off and block blood vessels in the lungs – the deep vein thrombosis that long-haul air travellers are warned about; and injecting the drug heparin to reduce the likelihood of blood clotting.

If there is a possibility that a patient will need blood, we are careful to ensure that it can be done quickly, so we take a sample the day before and find the closest match possible from the blood bank. On the end of every bag of blood there are what we call 'pigtails' – little straws with a small amount of blood in them – and we mix that with some of the patient's serum to make sure there isn't going to be a transfusion reaction. The process takes a few hours, so in trauma situations, where blood is needed urgently, we use standard O-negative, because it is the least likely to cause a problem.

We discuss the positioning of the patient on the operating table too, because sometimes we need to move them during the operation and that needs to be pre-planned. We also go through all the equipment and kit we will need, though to a varying degree the team members already have a pretty good idea of that from previous experiences. The equipment includes our standard kit of more than eighty instruments for every operation, plus the specific requirements for each one: for instance, what kind of saw we will need to cut through bones and what kind of tourniquet for any limbs from which we will be 'harvesting' tissue.

I then run through the standard checklist, immediately before we start operating. Is the patient diabetic? Does he need glycaemic (blood sugar) control? Is patient warming in place? Do we need to remove any hair from the body surface? Have antibiotics been administered? Does the patient have any allergies? If a blood transfusion is planned, has it been cross-matched? Is the blood available and in the fridge, ready for use? If it is going to be a long operation, I will also tell the staff that we will do our best to keep the whole team fresh, scrubbing out surgical staff at appropriate intervals, and making sure that everyone gets some food and water.

At the end of the briefing, enthused and ready to go in to bat for the patient, all the staff disperse to their respective stations to complete their own preparations, and one of the nurses calls the ward and asks for the patient to be brought down. My own next vitally important task is to sort out my music. On days when I'm operating I always have my own playlist with me. I have pop music for the early stages of the procedure and the close at the end, and more serious music – mainly, though not exclusively, classical music – for the technically demanding microsurgery phase that may last several hours.

Although there were a few CDs kicking around in most operating theatres early in my career, the soundtrack to a procedure was usually provided by the bleeping of the heart monitor. That sound always cuts through whatever music we have playing, but subconsciously you tend to blot it out in order to concentrate on other sounds around you that may have far greater significance.

Having said that, if its tone or pitch changes, you are instantly aware of it and on full alert.

I first had the opportunity to bring some of my own music into the operating theatre when I was a junior trainee in cardio-thoracic surgery. I slotted in *Moon Safari* by the French group Air, and as it began to play, the scrub nurse, a battle-hardened veteran of a thousand ops with a downturned mouth and a world-weary air, gave me a sideways look and said, in the broadest Glaswegian, 'So are you into aw that druggy music, then?' She then shrugged and carried on with what she was doing, but I didn't let her lack of enthusiasm put me off and kept on playing my own choice of music whenever I was operating. I still do during major surgery today. It's not just a personal quirk: there is solid scientific evidence that, when carrying out repetitive tasks requiring intense concentration, a surgeon's performance is improved and his anxiety levels are reduced if music he has personally selected is playing.

Music has also been shown to reduce anxiety in patients under local anaesthesia. There is even some evidence to suggest that those under general anaesthetic need less pain relief, both while asleep and afterwards, if music has been playing. In addition, music helps to reinforce the mood we always try to create at the pre-operative briefing: relaxed but focused and, if necessary, capable of swift and decisive action.

In non-major cases or in the early phases of a major operation, the soundtrack just needs to please everyone and avoid irritating anyone. A mixture of recent pop music, leaning more towards the Radio 2 playlist than Radio 1, often music from the 1980s, usually does the trick, but when we reach the microsurgery phase of the operation I feel the need to change the environment to one of quiet, focused concentration for the surgeons. That leaves nobody present in any doubt that we have reached a particularly demanding and technically challenging part of the procedure. Any visitors to the theatre suite then also benefit from an audio as well as a visual clue (the huge microscope that we use during microsurgery) that the cathedral-like atmosphere must not be disturbed.

Music has been important to me throughout my life and career, and not merely as a background soundtrack. Like all surgeons, I have to operate frequently to maintain my skills and technique and, unlike practising my flute, it is not a routine, two-hours-a-day process. However, playing the flute has also undoubtedly helped develop and hone my technical motor skills – my manual dexterity and delicacy of touch. I am convinced that the relentless practice I had to put in as a pupil learning the instrument when I was young not only made me a much better flute player, but a more skilful surgeon too. The technical stuff – scales and arpeggios – remains crucial to me even today. I still run through them the night before I'm in the operating theatre, and when I've done so, my hands will do what my mind wants them to more swiftly and efficiently during microsurgery and suturing than if I've just been sitting on the sofa watching television.

Like skilled musicians, surgeons need to make highly efficient use of their hands. Early in my surgical career I was struck by the fact that some of the consultants training me never seemed to rush, were always apparently relaxed and had very smooth and effective hand and finger movements. Now, when working with my own trainee surgeons, I always stress that it is not the speed at which you operate that counts, but the economy of movement you use, so that the surgery appears effortless.

The nicest compliment you can get is when someone says, 'You didn't seem to be rushing at all, but that's only taken twenty minutes.' During a recent procedure I overheard a student who was watching a senior fellow and me tying blood vessels whisper to his fellow student, 'It's like watching magic!' The key is thinking a few steps ahead: don't be rushing it, just make sure that every move is as efficient as possible. I am not saying that absolutely every movement counts and there is no redundancy at all, but you work to minimize that. It's a bit like a snooker player planning three or four shots ahead or a chess grandmaster visualizing checkmate several moves before he achieves it. The operation should look easy. If it looks like a struggle, it is probably because it wasn't planned well enough. It is also the best way to minimize difficulties and reduce operation time, which is very important in terms of patient outcomes – measured in free flap (transplanted tissue) survival rates, excellent wound healing, low rates of complications and above all, of course, the survival of the patient: the less time they spend anaesthetized and under the knife, the quicker and more complete will be their recovery afterwards.

Once our preparations are complete, with all the surgical team gloved, capped and gowned, and the surgeons and scrub nurses scrubbed-in, all the staff look anonymous, with only their eyes visible through the 'surgical letterbox' – the gap for the eyes between the cap and the top of the mask. All the sterile staff are also wearing either glasses or clear visors, to prevent spurting blood or other bodily fluids splashing into their eyes. It has often struck me that a surgical team can communicate remarkably well with just their eyes, especially when something has gone wrong and action is required. A narrowed glance, a widened eye, even a small gasp behind a mask can convey the most powerful message in the bright, hot, rarefied atmosphere of an operating theatre in full flow.

All the staff wearing exactly the same garb can make it a little confusing for those visitors I mentioned earlier – medical students, overseas guests or personnel from surgical device companies who are not scrubbed-in and observe from the periphery of the theatre, or from a viewing gallery if there is one. None of them will have a clue about anyone's seniority. The only hints might be a stray wisp of grey hair showing at the edge of someone's surgical hat, or the speed at which different surgeons suture because, confident in their skills and with years of training and practice behind them, consultants tend to suture much more quickly and accurately than registrars. Visitors can also find the trays of surgical instruments laid out ready for use quite bizarre-looking, even threatening, the array of bone saws, drills and retractors looking more like medieval torture implements than life-saving tools.

When the patient arrives from the ward, we make the final reconfirmation of his or her details and the procedure to be followed – the last stage of a triple checking process that ensures we are carrying out the correct operation on the correct patient. Mistakes have happened very occasionally in hospitals in the past, when a patient has been misidentified or has, for example, had an operation on his left arm when it should have been his right, so the exhaustive checks are there to make sure such errors never happen.

After the patient has been anaesthetized for a major operation, the first phase of the procedure, which we always hope to complete in half an hour, involves placing an arterial line into the artery at the patient's wrist, peripheral venous lines into the arms, and a central venous line deep in the neck. These allow us to precisely measure blood pressure from within the artery with every heartbeat, and safely deliver fluid and drugs. A tube is also fed down the throat into the windpipe, ensuring a safe airway, and a catheter is inserted into the bladder to measure urine output so we can monitor kidney function.

The unconscious patient is then wheeled through to the theatre and carefully positioned on the operating table. This is a complex team manoeuvre, requiring great care to avoid dislodging the numerous lines and tubes that are keeping him safe. He has a foam blanket underneath him to keep him warm and gel packs are also placed at pressure points under him to keep him comfortable and still. To keep his whole body warm, he is covered by a 'Bair Hugger', because anaesthetized patients can't regulate their own core temperature and even a 1° drop doubles the risk of infection. A Bair Hugger is a single-use blanket with micro-perforations through which heated air is blown; a forced-air warming system that prevents hypothermia and other complications during surgery, such as increased rate of infection and higher blood loss. The patient's body is also covered in sterile blue surgical sheets, held in place by steel scissor clamps, with just the sites to be operated on left exposed. Many surgeons say they prefer to have their patients' faces covered during operations, making the procedure more neutral and impersonal for them rather than having a constant reminder of the individual they are treating in front of them, but of course that is not a luxury a maxillofacial surgeon can ever enjoy.

I don't really get butterflies before carrying out a procedure any more, but I am like an athlete on the starting blocks, wound up, waiting for the gun to fire . . . so there is nothing more frustrating than a delayed start or, worse, a postponement. That's a very rare event, though – in the Institute for Neurological Sciences in Glasgow perhaps twice a year across the three major facial surgery teams. And I can recall only one occurrence in the three years I spent at the Royal Marsden and Northwick Park hospitals in London. When I worked in the Bradford Teaching Hospitals in Yorkshire delays were more frequent, usually a wait for the ITU (Intensive Treatment Unit) ward round to be completed. That was not the fault of any staff, though: the delays were usually caused because an ITU patient who was ready to be moved to another ward, thus freeing up an ITU bed, had to stay where she was because a patient well enough to go to social care could not leave the destination ward because there was nowhere for him to go. This sort of thing happened at least twice a month – very frustrating for everybody concerned. But postponements, again, were mercifully rare, only once every four to six months.

Once we're ready to go, the first surgical step is always to replace the tube down the patient's throat with an airway, a tracheostomy breathing tube surgically placed in his neck. The next step is to carry out an EUA (Examination Under Anaesthesia) – a detailed inspection with the patient asleep on the operating table. In an operation to excise a tumour, for example, the EUA determines the exact area of facial tissue that is to be removed. We use a special stain containing iodine to precisely delineate the cancerous and pre-cancerous tissue, thereby minimizing the impairment of the patient's appearance, and his speech and ability to swallow.

Many of our operations involve a 'free flap transfer': a piece of human tissue – skin, flesh, muscle and sometimes bone – cut out of one of a number of different sites around the body and then transplanted into a different site to remedy a defect that may be congenital, or caused by trauma, or the excision of a tumour. Bone from the shoulder-blade, hip or fibula can be used to reconstruct the jaw, while skin and soft tissue from the arm or thigh can form a new tongue or the floor of the mouth. We measure the exact size and volume of the void that will be left after the tumour has been removed, which tells us precisely how much tissue we will need for reconstruction from elsewhere in the body. We write it all down and draw the shape to the same scale on the whiteboard in the operating theatre, so we can use it as the template for the free flap (the area of tissue we are going to transplant). We draw very accurate lines on the skin with purple skin-marking ink, precisely placing the incision lines over the shape and size of tissue required, and centring over the underlying blood vessels that supply that area of tissue.

As always when operating, as I prepare to make the first incision there is a moment of anticipation when time seems to slow down and I become hyper-aware of every sight, sound and sensation: the music playing quietly; the monotone beeping of the heart monitor; the sound of the suction device – like a muted vacuum cleaner – which changes to a 'slooshing' noise as excess blood and other fluids begin to be sucked away; the whirring of the extractor fans; and even the faint feeling of air movement against the exposed skin around my eyes. I still feel a frisson of excitement as I anticipate the familiar sight of the surgical blade parting the skin surface, exposing the yellow subcutaneous fat and, beneath it, the sheen of the silvery fascia that covers the red-brown muscles. The incision is as clean as a drawn line on paper for an instant, and then bright crimson blood begins oozing from the severed edges and seeping into the surgical cut. At this point there is an almost overwhelming sense of entering into a sanctuary, where nothing can distract from the purpose at hand and there is total focus on the person lying in front of me. A hospital is the only building in the world where no one moves when the fire alarm goes off.

Although the incisions are precise, newcomers to the operating theatre are always surprised by the amount of physical force that is needed to cut through human skin, or peel back neck skin and muscle tissues. We tend to imagine that our skin and flesh are quite delicate, but they're much tougher than we think and it takes a real effort to pull them back to expose an underlying structure.

There is sometimes a faint smell as the flesh opens which registers on your subconscious as much as your conscious mind, because you are focusing so hard on the procedure, but there is little sound, unless you're using a laser or a Colorado diathermy needle instead of a scalpel. The Colorado needle is a monopolar electrode that burns through tissue using high-frequency shortwave electric current at its incredibly sharp tungsten tip. It makes a faint buzzing noise each time you cut with it, and the act of cutting also produces a musical note. The needle also has another setting to make blood vessels coagulate and that produces a different note, with the two notes a minor third apart, like Brahms' Lullaby. Every time I hear those notes it feels like a slightly disconcerting juxtaposition to me, given that what we're doing at that point would be most unlikely to lull anyone to sleep.

Using the Colorado needle also generates puffs of smoke which have to be suctioned away because they may contain viral particles. You can smell the burnt flesh when you're using it, and sometimes when you walk into the operating theatre suite you can instantly tell that a hip replacement or some other major surgery has been going on, because you're assaulted by a smell like the aroma of a bad barbecue.

When I have completed the excision of the tumour with a good margin around it to eliminate any microscopic cancer spread, I turn my attention to the lymph nodes in the patient's neck. Partly as a result of a huge randomized controlled trial in India, it has now been established that even if there is no detectable sign of cancer there, removing the lymph nodes is life-saving for the 20 or 30 per cent of patients who already have an invisible microscopic cancer spread to the neck. So I next expose the outer surface of the shiny yellow envelope of tissue that contains the lymphatic vessels and lymph nodes, lying beneath the platysma muscle in the neck, distinctively marked by vertical stripes at intervals. I dissect this layer free from the muscles and blood vessels using scalpels and scissors and a new device called a harmonic scalpel. This looks like a *Star Wars* version of scissors, but uses ultrasonic vibration to separate and simultaneously seal human tissue, and can remarkably reduce the oozing of blood when tissue is cut.

Removing the lymph glands in the neck also gives us access to the blood vessels in the carotid arteries to which we will attach the transplanted tissue flap. The priority when I'm doing a neck dissection is to remove the lymph glands and the disease they may contain but equally to make sure I leave the neck with a beautiful (usually facial) artery and a perfectly prepared internal jugular vein. These will accommodate the flap of transplanted tissue and connect with the tiny blood vessels, only two to three millimetres in diameter, that will supply oxygenated blood to the flap and drain it. Like a lot of things in life, the best time to get all this right is the first time. If we prepare and plan meticulously, with all the blood vessels the right length, all lined up, and the vessels in the neck sitting passively and perfectly, then the subsequent microsurgery to connect them to the free flap should not be difficult and complex.

Another technique we use to make free tissue reconstruction more reliable is to base the flap on 'perforating vessels' – the very tiny arteries and veins that run up to and down to the skin surface from the large blood vessels that we use in the arms, legs and trunk. Although we can predict where these are likely to be, we will make the first incision so we have a choice of where to harvest the skin for a flap, and so can have the perforating vessels sitting right in the middle of the tissue we transplant. This is personalized medicine, custom-tailored to the anatomy of our patient.

While I'm working on the facial surgery, another surgeon will be preparing to harvest the bone and tissue for the free flap to reconstruct the face and neck. Having two surgeons, one preparing the flap to be transplanted while the other one excises the tumour and prepares the site to receive the flap, greatly reduces the duration of the operation and therefore the risk that fatigue in the surgeons or the medical team will lead to errors. It also cuts the amount of time the patient has to remain under anaesthesia, which in turn reduces the time needed for him to recover from the operation. Each of us also has a trainee surgeon assisting and observing us, learning the skills that will ultimately enable them to take the lead role themselves.

All the time we are operating, the sounds of the theatre include the constant murmur of nurses counting aloud. Everything we use is counted in and counted out again and everything must be accounted for. It's done to ensure that no small instruments, swabs or anything else are left inside the patient, and the count is always carried out in a particular way. When I have finished with a swab, for example, I will pass it back (sometimes requesting 'Another one of these in white') or simply drop it on to the sheet covering the patient's body. The scrub nurse picks it up with her tongs and throws it into a stainless steel bowl and one of the non-sterile nurses then picks it up with her tongs and puts it in one of the pockets of a clear plastic sheet – like a transparent advent calendar – hanging on the wall of the operating theatre. When it's full, it is discarded and a fresh one hung up. One of the staff nurses counts the number of used swabs out loud in front of another nurse who then makes her own count of them, and the total is compared to the number of clean swabs that have been issued.

It is a vital procedure and is treated with absolute care and seriousness, because if those numbers do not match at the end of the operation and all other possible explanations have been ruled out, the assumption will be that a swab has been left in the patient, who will then have to be reopened in search of it. None of us is ever complacent about it because a mislaid swab could have fatal consequences for the patient. It has never yet happened in one of my operations, though we once had a very close call. At the end of a major operation but before we began to close the patient, we discovered that a swab was missing and neither myself nor my colleague could believe it was inside the patient. Yet we followed the didactic theatre protocol and X-rayed the patient (swabs have a thick radio-opaque thread in them so show up clearly on an X-ray) and there it was, nestling in the very root of the neck, hiding behind the big muscles, like a small medical IED ready to sabotage our patient and our work.

When we have completed the resection (cutting out) of the tumour, we send a tiny piece of the surrounding tissue to the pathologist. If we've left any tumour cells behind there – and on the CT and MRI imaging we have, it is always quite hard to tell how far the cancer has spread – then the cancer will recur from that point. If it is in the bone, then even radiotherapy will be of no help.

While the sample is being snap-frozen in the lab and then examined under the microscope, we have a breather, a bite to eat and take on some fluid. Before we do so, the theatre staff dress the patient with saline-soaked swabs to restrict the loss of fluid from his body through evaporation. For dignity's sake they also cover his face with some surgical drapes, and then leave him asleep, stable and comfortable, and watched over by the anaesthetic team monitoring his vital signs.

When the lab report comes back, hopefully negative, and everyone has been fed and watered and had a few minutes' rest, we go back into the theatre. The free flap for the reconstruction is all but detached, apart from the artery supplying blood and the vein draining it. We clamp and divide them, securely tying the stumps of the blood vessels left behind, and the instant that we do so I call 'Flap off!' and our theatre healthcare assistant writes the 'detach time' on one of the theatre whiteboards. For obvious reasons, even though we are still working in the same calm and unhurried way, we aim to keep the time that the flap remains detached from a blood supply to an absolute minimum.

Once I am satisfied that the free flap is an absolutely perfect fit for the space left by the removal of the tumour – and I continue to shape and sculpt it until I am – everything is in readiness for the complex part of the procedure. This is the point at which the large microscope we use in microsurgery is wheeled up to the table. German-made (Zeiss) and generally thought to be the best on the market, it is a huge and very heavy machine, around eight feet tall with a base about three feet square, but so beautifully engineered – *Vorsprung durch Technik!* – and so perfectly balanced that it feels as light as a feather when we're adjusting it. There's a pair of periscope eyepieces each for the surgeon and his assistant (either another consultant or a trainee surgeon, sitting on the other side of the patient's head), and the view down the scope is binocular – both eyes – so depth perception is clear. There are buttons for zoom and focus like a computer gaming device, and another button to release and move the microscope head. A light click resets the scope, so the surgeon can set the eyepieces to his own inter-pupillary distance (that is, the distance between the pupils of his eyes – in my case 61.5mm). There are also plus and minus rings around the eyepiece, to adjust depth of field.

The arrival of this huge piece of technology feels like a metaphor for the extreme technical phase we are now entering. I feel a further surge of excitement and focused relaxation as I arrange myself on the microsurgery chair. I make small adjustments to its arms until they are the perfect height for me to rest my elbows and relax my shoulders, while leaving my hands completely free to make tiny movements with my fingers. I exhale in a long sigh that always precedes the controlled breathing once I begin microsurgery in the bright, vivid view before my eyes, with the gentle beep of the circulating blood registering faintly in my subconscious. This is now the inner sanctum.

At the same time as the microscope is brought up to the operating table, we switch to the serious music. My playlist for this phase of the procedure, which can last several hours, includes film scores and piano works by the Scottish composer Craig Armstrong, but is mostly baroque: Bach, Handel, some Vivaldi and Alessandro Marcello. There is also some beautiful Vaughan Williams (*Fantasia on a Theme by Thomas Tallis*) and, by way of contrast, a cheeky *Braveheart* theme – practically de rigueur for a Scottish surgeon when working south of Hadrian's Wall. The baroque selection in particular – flute sonatas and piano music such as *The Goldberg Variations* – for me imparts a structure and a sense of tangible discipline to the environment. The selected recordings are classic virtuoso performances, full of lyricism and enormous musicality, and that is a great metaphor for the process of surgical reconstruction because, while it has to be technically perfect, there is also room for differences of approach and interpretation. For example, I have found that in some parts of the human body a gentle elliptical skin excision often leaves a less obvious scar than a straight line. Surgery is an art as well as a science.

As soon as the serious music begins, everything becomes absolutely calm, quiet and relaxed. The atmosphere is helped by dimming the main lights over the operating table. The brilliant light they give is necessary during other phases of the operation, but the microscope for microsurgery has its own integral lights, so the rest are switched off, leaving the operating theatre in relative darkness.

As I operate, the scrub nurse stands alongside me, watching every moment of the procedure on a high-definition LCD monitor and handing me each instrument as I ask for it. Scrub nurses – men and women – are highly skilled and know the exact location of the up to 180 different instruments on their tray so intimately that as soon as I ask for one of them – and if something has gone wrong, I won't be wanting it in thirty seconds, I'll be wanting it right now – they can instantly pick it up and slap it in my hand. They are often even quicker than that: so experienced are they, and so closely are they following what I am doing, they are able to anticipate my requirements almost before I am aware of them myself, and even as I am beginning to form the words they have already selected the instrument and are putting it in my hand.

While the scrub nurse follows the procedure on her monitor, another screen relays the images from the microscope so that everyone else in the theatre can also see what is going on. That, too, reinforces the message that we are into a quiet phase of the operation. Even so, there have been a few occasions in the past when I have had to ask people in the theatre to be quiet, because sometimes there can be two or three new people on the team, or observing the procedure, who have not yet learned the rules. It is partly a matter of respect for the patient and the technical difficulty of microsurgery, but silence is also particularly important if a trainee is doing the procedure, because the aim is to build their confidence, not erode it, and it can be very difficult to focus on the extreme microscopic task if there's too much distracting extraneous noise.

Eyes glued to the microscope, I start to prepare the ends of the minute artery for the free flap. I take away the elastic tissue adventitia (the outside layer) and prepare it – but without over-preparing it – by sharp dissection with micro-scissors and tiny forceps (the ones used by watchmakers and jewellers). I also have to ensure that the inside of the blood vessel is in good condition because, particularly with people who have smoked a lot – and that accounts for the majority of head and neck cancer patients – the intima (inside lining) can become detached, leading to blood clots. That is always very bad news, because clotting inside the tiny blood vessels supplying and draining the flap will lead to the death of the reconstruction tissue, more major surgery and a very difficult, gaping wound to manage.

Sometimes the blood vessels can be of such poor quality that it is like trying to sew together two damp cornflakes, and if we are unsuccessful in connecting them because of their condition we have to prepare them again after cutting them back to a shorter length. If we have been meticulous and have taken ten minutes longer on the neck dissection to make sure we have plenty of length in the neck artery to which we attach the transplanted tissue, we have several chances to cut back to a part of the vessel in better condition, but if we only give ourselves one shot and it doesn't work, we are in serious trouble . . . and so is the patient.

We attach the artery taken from the donor site to the facial artery in the neck with sutures that are almost invisible to the naked eye. An artery three millimetres in diameter requires nine to twelve sutures, and just occasionally while sewing them we can lose the tiny, curved, stainless steel needle at the tip of the jeweller forceps we are using, because it can ping out and disappear from the microscope field. They're so minute that they can't really do any harm, but of course we would never knowingly leave one in a patient.

If we do lose one, despite a search with the microscope around the operating field, we have to complete an incident report. One ophthalmic surgeon was so annoyed at having to do so when he lost one of those tiny needles on the floor of the operating theatre that he wrote to the general manager of the hospital: 'I'm sorry you feel I have to fill out a full incident form every time I lose one of these tiny sutures. They are really tiny, you see, and very difficult to identify if they ping out of view on to the floor. In fact I've put one in this envelope, so you can see for yourself.' And of course he didn't put one in the envelope . . .

When we have successfully attached the artery from the donor site to the artery supplying blood to the patient's face and completed the sutures, we release the micro-clamps, allowing the artery to flow and fill the flap with oxygen-carrying blood. I call 'Flap on!' and the theatre assistant works out the 'ischaemic time' – the period that the flap has gone without blood flow and oxygen supply, ideally well under an hour. The blood vessels then fill and pulse, expanding and vibrating, giving a sense of reanimation – new life for this part of the face.

We then attach the flap vein to the neck vein, this time with even smaller stitches that are invisible to the naked eye, and as an additional safeguard we attach a Doppler microprobe to it, an early warning system that generates a *whoosh whoosh* sound when blood is flowing past the microsurgical join in the vessels. Virtually the whole team tend to cluster around the tiny Doppler box, listening for the tell-tale sounds that let us know the flap is functioning correctly. No sound equals no blood flow, and that means the flap will fail, so we will have to try again.

Normal blood pressure is about 120 over 80, but when we're taking out a tumour or raising a free flap, I ask the anaesthetist to reduce the patient's blood pressure to minimize blood loss and it can be as low as 90 over 60. Later in the operation, when we have transferred the tissue and I want the free flap to perfuse with blood, I ask the anaesthetist to increase the flow so the pressure rises again. Although it's a liquid, blood usually consists of 55 per cent cells, and the fewer cells it contains, the faster it will flow. So to improve blood flow through a transplanted flap, we will allow a patient to bleed down from a higher haemoglobin count of as much as 160 grams per litre to about 100, by simply not replacing lost blood. Patients bleed from their surgically created wounds, so the amount of blood we elect to replace dictates the haemoglobin count (the stuff carrying vital oxygen), and if the patient is slightly anaemic, the blood is less viscous and will flow through the transplanted tissue more easily, paradoxically delivering more vital oxygen, not less.

We let the flap run for ten or fifteen minutes to be certain all is well before we begin to close. Patience at this point can be as important as swift and efficient operating at other times during major surgery: this is not the time to be rushing out of the building. Occasionally the reconstruction will look good, but when we place the microprobe on the micro-vein there will be no signal, and we'll know there is still something we need to fix.

With the microsurgery phase complete, we are through the most intense part of the operation and, after working for several hours, we have now reached the end-game. From that point, ninety-nine times out of a hundred we will be able to close the operated sites, scrub out and be heading for home within a couple of hours. So as usual we change the music to a more upbeat, feel-good closing playlist, designed to lift the spirits and breathe life into the tired minds and limbs of the operating team, though the volume always needs to be turned down at this point. After the stately, measured rhythms of Bach or Handel, a sudden, explosive guitar riff can be a shock to the system – the sort of shock a surgeon holding a razor-sharp scalpel should avoid at all costs.

We check again that everything is running well and there are still no alarm signals from the Doppler microprobes, and then we start to close. To prevent a build-up of fluid, we begin placing drains – silicone tubes attached to razor sharp 'trochars' (spikes) which push through the neck skin and are secured with black silk sutures – into the patient's neck, allowing fluid to escape and aiding the healing process. There is a palpably lighter atmosphere in the room now: we are heading for the home straight with this patient.

When we close the area from which the flap has been harvested, we put the incised edges together and sew them. If possible, we stretch the surrounding skin over the area, but quite often it needs a skin graft too, an extra piece of free skin which we usually take from the abdomen – so my patients often get a small tummy tuck at no extra charge!

Once the close is complete, I write up the record of the operation with one of the registrars, and it has to be meticulously compiled. All the pathology specimens (the pieces of excised body tissue that are sent off for examination) have to be labelled, and often we have to make some adjustment to them, because tissue is elastic and can shrink by as much as 25 per cent after removal from the body and processing in the lab. Bits of the removed tissue can also move around, so it is vital to reposition these precisely, just as they were in the patient's face. If the pathologists section the pieces we have removed when they have shrunk after being preserved in formalin, they may get a false reading, suggesting that we have had what we call a 'close margin' and may not have cleared a wide enough area around the cancerous tissue to be confident of a cure. As a result, we always prepare the tumour tissue carefully to be sure that the pathologists' measurements under their microscope are an accurate reflection of the size and orientation of the tissue when we removed it from the patient. When we are excising a tumour, that care can mean sparing the patient other treatments such as radiotherapy or chemotherapy which, while they may eradicate the remaining cancer, will also cause permanent damage to the recipient's body.

While we are writing up the records, the still-unconscious patient is in the process of being transferred from the operating table to a hospital bed. With all the lines, tubes, catheters and wires still attached to him, this is far from a straightforward task and takes about eight highly experienced staff to complete. As soon as he is in place, the nurses elevate the head-end of the bed to between 30° and 45°, because the effect of gravity reduces venous pressure in the head and neck, thereby lessening the likelihood of swelling and bleeding. The nurses check that all the readings are still normal and stable (stable simply means unchanging), and then announce, 'Obs [observations] OK.' That is the point at which we can all really start to relax.

*

The patient is moved to the Intensive Care Unit (ICU) or High Dependency Unit (HDU) – the location depending on the particular patient and procedure we have carried out – where he can be closely monitored by specialist nursing staff and kept warm, comfortable and pain-free overnight. After a long anaesthetic and operation, patients can take some time to sleep off the effects and regain consciousness, so we switch off the sedative drugs as soon as they are installed in the HDU to help them wake up and begin to breathe spontaneously again. The reason for that is there is much less chance of a chest infection if the lungs are properly aerated, as they are during natural breathing. A ventilator is considerably less effective at doing that: if a patient is kept on a ventilator for more than twenty-four hours, the risk of pneumonia increases dramatically.

When we wake them, our patients are never looking at their best, with a swollen face and neck (though with very neat scars) and sometimes the beginnings of bruise marks from the surgery. By the following morning they might look even worse, with more swelling and bruising, but after a couple of days have passed, any bruised tissues are changing colour from blue and purple to a yellow tinge as they begin to fade.

My patients are not usually compos mentis when I make my immediate post-op visit, but whether or not they remember it afterwards, I always try to reassure them that the trauma has been worthwhile. So I always speak to them as people, very directly. I stand beside their beds and tell them, 'Everything's fine. The operation couldn't have gone better.' Sometimes I don't get any response at all, sometimes it's just a grunt or a few random words from the dream I've just interrupted, but I hope the message penetrates and helps them to get an untroubled natural sleep later on. This is a blissful time for the surgeon, who is filled with a sense of achievement after a difficult job well done, coupled with a certain numb tiredness. I often notice hospital sounds and smells more at these times.

I always have the phone number for the next of kin and, so it doesn't get lost, I usually write it on the consent form signed by the patient or, in the case of a minor, his legal guardian, along with the security question that they've been prepared for, usually something like 'Where did you and I first meet?' I can then phone them straight after the operation and reassure them that everything has gone well – and, as I said, ninety-nine times out of a hundred it has. That's one of the best phone calls you can ever make, because you can feel the sense of relief and joy at the other end of the phone.

However, sometimes the feeling that comes through from the patient's family is more a sort of numbness. The relatives have been under so much stress and tension, and have expended so much nervous energy in the build-up to the operation, that when the worst is at last over and we phone them with the good news, the entire process they have been through can just make them drained and devoid of any apparent emotion – though obviously that is not how they will be feeling inside.

My next mission is to drink a couple of litres of water because I always have to rehydrate after a long day in the operating theatre, where the temperature is warm enough to guarantee the comfort of the patient and therefore the discomfort of the surgical and medical staff. In order to avoid transmission of potentially harmful fluids from patient to surgeon, we also wear impervious gowns made from material that does not breathe well, and which make us overheat even more. My watch begins the day strapped tight around my wrist, but on operating days it is often sliding around on my forearm by the evening.

Once I am sure that everything is fine with my patient, I am free to leave the hospital, but after a long day in theatre I often don't head home straight away and instead take the surgical team to the pub across the road for a debrief and a chat over a drink, maybe a single beer. The process of reflection after significant events is well established in medicine and forms part of the post-surgery process. If one of the trainees has done a good job, I'll make a point of telling them so, because the whole point is to give the trainees not just the skills but also the confidence to lead a surgical team themselves in due course.

However, by the same token, if mistakes happen, for whatever reason, they need to be addressed. Many senior surgeons have a reputation for not suffering fools, but feedback needs to be a careful, thorough and respectful process. My trainees are never criticized in public; the feedback process takes place in private, and even then the discussion of the outcomes will be balanced, positive criticism. Even the most qualified and experienced of us should not be exempt from constructive criticism. I have to be able to say to one of my colleagues, and they have to be able to say to me, 'That could have gone better,' or, better still, 'Tell you what, you tell me how you thought that went,' because self-reflection and self-evaluation are vital to any surgeon or other medical professional. If we don't do it, we don't improve.

It is just as important, of course, to acknowledge the contribution of the team members when things are going well, and it is a great feeling to sit around together after a major operation, sharing that quiet sense of achievement. If a complex reconstruction doesn't work, it's devastating – all that surgery of the tumour site and the donor site (where the reconstruction tissue is taken from) wasted; but the benefits when it does work, which is almost every time, are tremendous. When we do get it right, it is deeply satisfying. But just occasionally something will creep in and bite us on the backside. That is always a timely reminder, making us realize not how precarious but how sensitive are the techniques we use, every little bit of them. Ours is a precise science, of course, but it is also a kind of multi-disciplinary alchemy, and I always experience a slight sense of wonder at the end of a major operation: how could that possibly have all worked out so that a patient with a potentially fatal disease has been restored to a full and healthy life again?

2

AS I WALKED into my consulting rooms one bright spring morning, my first patient was already waiting. Faisal was a fourteen-year-old boy, a promising swimmer who had first come to see me, accompanied by his parents, a few weeks before. At six feet he was very tall for his age and, as teenagers can be, he had initially appeared to be quite cocky, but the way he caught his lower lip between his teeth in unguarded moments suggested that he was less composed than he wanted people to believe.

His father, wearing a business suit, had been an immigrant to the UK from Kashmir. He'd done most of the talking at first, explaining what had brought them to me. Faisal's mother, a second-generation Briton whose parents were also of Asian origin, wore traditional dress and said almost nothing to begin with, though her eyes never left her son and her concern for him was etched in every line on her face.

The boy had a large, disfiguring swelling on the jaw, caused by a tumour in his mandible that was giving rise to increasing physical discomfort and was also affecting his confidence – always a fragile commodity in an adolescent. His father told me that the lump had started as a painless swelling on the right-side, lower-third of Faisal's face but it had now become very sore and was also occasionally bleeding into the boy's mouth.

His father went on to explain the background to the case, and why it had taken seven weeks for the relevant paperwork to be passed along the chain to me. That was unacceptable because we have a protocol that if a doctor suspects a patient has cancer, they can send us a pro-forma which requires us to see the patient within fourteen days – and once they are in front of me, I can get a CT scan (often in thirty minutes) and a biopsy a few minutes after that, which will show exactly what we are dealing with. But this had not happened in Faisal's case. He had first been seen by a registrar who did not prioritize his biopsy – it was processed as 'non-urgent' – and information about him was not passed to me. The delay in being referred to me had only made matters worse for him.

Faisal's X-ray showed a tumour that was multi-locular (consisting of a number of small compartments or cells), but from the imaging we had it was not possible to tell if it was benign or malignant, so as a first step we took a biopsy, using two large samples out of the lower jawbone, in order to establish what we were dealing with. The findings would tell us whether we could simply excise the tumour or if we'd need to remove a whole section of his lower jaw with the surrounding soft tissue, and replace it with a free flap of transplanted tissue from his leg, forearm or abdomen.

The results from the lab confirmed that it was an ameloblastoma, a type of benign tumour formed from tooth-forming precursor cells and thus more common in children than adults. Even though they are rarely malignant (truly invading and destroying local tissue, and spreading to other body sites), they are locally aggressive – growing into the surrounding muscles, skin and mucous membranes – and, if not removed with a wide margin of normal tissue, they will come back, often years later.

Moreover, when they do recur, it is often as multiple tumours spread through the face, which can be difficult to treat well. In Faisal's case, to make sure that we removed all traces of the cancer, I calculated that we were going to have to cut out nine centimetres of his mandible, along with the attached facial muscles and mouth lining.

As gently as I could, I began to outline the necessary surgery and reconstruction, and explained the risks involved.

'To fix this, we need to remove the lump from here to here,' I said, tracing a line along Faisal's jaw with my finger.

Not surprisingly, the boy's bravado started to evaporate. 'What?' His voice had risen an octave.

'And remove part of either your fibula or your hip, and one layer of the wall of your tummy—'

'Whaaat?!'

'—to reconstruct this side of your face and mouth.'

In the space of a few minutes he moved from cocky teenager whose expression seemed to say 'You can't tell me anything, because you're a dad' to looking absolutely shattered at the prospect of what was to come.

'How long is all that going to take?' Faisal said.

'About seven hours,' I replied, keeping my voice steady, trying to hold his gaze in a way that was confident but not challenging. At times like this my Glaswegian accent often seems to help, perhaps making me seem a slightly less remote, aloof figure than someone speaking pure 'Home Counties English'.

Faisal lowered his eyes and stared at the floor for the first time. I could sense the information sinking in, like a court sentence being passed and digested. My aim now was to build up his sense of security and confidence in the surgical team, and in the next stages of the process. His parents had also been listening intently to every second of our conversation, absorbing every detail, and I needed to gain their confidence and trust as well.

'But do you know what, Faisal?' I continued. 'You're going to be an easy day at the office for us.'

He gave me a puzzled look. 'Really? Why? What do you mean?'

'Well, our patients are usually a lot older than you, and are often not in the best physical condition, or unwell for a whole load of other reasons apart from the cancer itself. They may be overweight, or heavy smokers or drinkers, or suffering from all sorts of degenerative diseases, and many of them will not have taken any serious exercise since they left school forty or fifty years before. We hardly ever have a young, promising athlete under our care. In fact, you might well be the fittest patient we have ever operated on.'

When I said that, I could at once see some of the tension seeping out of his shoulder muscles, and as we continued talking, I began to realize that the health risks, the potential impact of the surgery, the facial reconstruction, and the possibility that the cancer might recur were not his most significant worries. After his initial shock, with the adaptability of youth he'd quickly got used to the idea of those, and the only thing he really wanted to know from me now was, 'How fast am I going to be able to get back in the pool?'

I'd been a competitive swimmer myself at university, and I compared notes on times and training methods with him before telling him that, if all went well, I hoped we would have him back in the water within two to three months.

His eyes widened. 'Really?'

'I don't see why not.'

As they left my office, I was pleased to see that all three of them looked a lot more positive about the outcome than when I'd first broken the news to them.

Now that I knew just how important swimming was to Faisal, I kept that firmly in mind as I began planning the operation. As a result, the first decision I made was not to take the bone graft to reconstruct his jaw from the fibula in his leg – the thinnest of all the long bones of the body, running alongside the tibia (shinbone) on the outside of the calf. My knowledge of anatomy coupled with my own experience as a competitive swimmer had taught me that, although the power of the freestyle kick comes from big muscles in the pelvis and the top of the leg, the ankle needs to be relaxed enough to allow for efficient propulsion through the water. If we replaced a section of his jawbone with bone and skin from his fibula, as we might well have done in other circumstances, the resulting stiffness further down the leg would have slowed him down in the water.

Instead I decided that we would use his iliac crest, the section of bone on the outside of the pelvis – when you put your hands on your hips, you're resting them on the iliac crest. It would make an excellent replacement for part of the jaw because, rotated through 90°, the curve of the pelvis is very similar to the curve of the mandible.

I explained the logic of taking the transplant to rebuild his mandible from there at my final pre-op meeting with Faisal and his parents, so my visit to the ward on the morning of his operation was really just a chance to see him in a calm environment and reassure him that everything was going to be OK before he was brought down to the operating theatre.

'We're all set, Faisal,' I said. 'I've got a great team working with me and everything is going to be fine. So I'll see you back on the ward in a few hours' time.'

A little of his old cockiness resurfaced. 'Sure, whatever,' he said. 'See you later, doc.' But his voice betrayed him, cracking a little as he said it.

When Faisal was brought down from the ward, we made the final reconfirmation of all his details and the procedure that we would be carrying out. He was then anaesthetized, wheeled through to the operating theatre and positioned on the operating table. We first did the examination under anaesthesia to exactly determine the area of his jawbone and the surrounding tissue of his mouth and face that we would be removing: the less healthy tissue we took away, the less the damage to Faisal's appearance and oral functions – chewing, swallowing and speaking – that we would have to repair and rebuild.

We measured the exact size and volume of the void that would be left after the tumour had been removed from his jaw, which told us precisely how much bone, skin and fascia (the layer between the thin surface skin and the underlying muscles) from his hip and abdomen we would need for reconstruction, and drew the outlines in purple ink on his skin.

We raised Faisal's neck flap below the platysma muscle in the neck, and separated the tissue containing the lymph nodes and lymphatic vessels from the surrounding flesh and muscle, using the harmonic scalpel to minimize bleeding. We then approached the lower jawbone at the top of the operation site. It was gleaming white and solid-looking, but bulging in places, egg-shell thin, with the menacing purple tumour mass just below the fragile, expanded surface. I carefully stripped the soft tissue from the mandibular bone a full centimetre from where the tumour stopped on our scans, then began to cut through the jawbone. The saw blade made a buzzing sound and the vibrations ran up my arms as the blade cut unerringly through the healthy bone. I slowed the blade as the cut neared completion, hearing a final *click* as the bone ends parted, leaving fresh blood oozing from the healthy bone marrow. I made another precisely planned saw-cut at the back of the lower jaw, and the tumour-invaded bone now sat free.

We then removed some of the tissue from inside the cut bone ends with a bone curette, a small surgical instrument like an ice-cream scoop, and sent it to the laboratory to check for tumour cells. Having completed the excision of the tumour with a good margin around it to eliminate any spread that was too microscopic to be seen on our imaging, we turned our attention to the lymph nodes in Faisal's neck, dissected them out and then prepared the neck vein and artery ready to receive the transplanted free flap.

While we were doing that, Abdul, a younger and very skilled consultant surgeon, who also had a trainee surgeon assisting and observing him, was harvesting the bone and tissue for the flap. Abdul first made an oblique incision in the right side of Faisal's stomach and then deepened it on to the outer layer of muscle wall, which he divided to remove the middle layer of muscle, still attached to the hip bone. He traced and carefully dissected out the deep circumflex iliac artery and vein – the blood vessels supplying and draining this area – and finally used a bone saw to make cuts and remove a piece of bone from the iliac crest that was similar in shape to the section of the lower jaw we were removing. He left this flap with its muscles and other soft tissue still attached to Faisal's circulation until we had completed the careful excision of the tumour from his face and the removal of the lymph glands from his neck.

We were now almost four hours into the operation, and while waiting for the test results to come back from the lab we took a breather, had a snack and drank some water, leaving Faisal under his Bair Hugger, warm and asleep, but still watched over by the consultant anaesthetist and a member of the nursing team.

To my relief, the lab report was negative – no trace of tumour spread in the surrounding tissue – so we trooped back into theatre to prepare for the next, vital phase. We clamped and cut the last items connecting the free flap for Faisal's reconstruction to its original site, the artery supplying blood and the vein draining it, and tied off the stumps of those blood vessels. The free flap was now living up to its name, and I called 'Flap off!' so that our theatre healthcare assistant, Bhindhi, could write the detach time on the whiteboard.

We checked that the flap was the right size and shape to fill the void in Faisal's face, jaw and neck, and then spent some time sculpting the new jawbone and soft tissues to ensure an absolutely perfect fit, guaranteeing that his appearance, speech and ability to swallow would be fully restored. We shaped and sculpted the bone with surgical chisels and a mallet, and a large burr (drill-bit) attached to a motorized handpiece. Once his transplanted flap had healed into the facial site and settled down after the surgery, Faisal would also need to have a prosthesis fitted to replace the teeth he had lost when we removed that section of his jaw.

The Zeiss 88 microscope was then wheeled up to the table

and we switched to the serious-music playlist. As usual, the atmosphere changed at once, from the bright lights and busy bustle of the early stages of the operation to an almost cathedral-like quiet, and with the main operating theatre lights dimmed, the pool of light cast by the microscope centred everyone's attention. My whole focus was on the view through the eye-pieces of the microscope as we prepared the ends of the tiny artery to connect the free flap. It was a much less stressful procedure than in many cases, because Faisal was young, fit and healthy, and his blood vessels were in excellent condition. Even so, as we attached the flap to his jaw, it was essential to leave room for a little 'give' by allowing a gentle curve for the pedicle (the ribbon-shaped bit with the blood vessels in it), though not so much that the thin-walled vessels would stretch and tear if Faisal turned his head. We sutured it down with a slightly bigger stitch, to make sure it sat perfectly. As with most phases of the procedure, the margins between success and failure were very fine, but drawing on years of experience, the judgement I employ has become largely instinctive.

We attached the artery taken from Faisal's pelvis to the facial artery in his neck with microscopic sutures. That went perfectly, and once we'd completed the suturing, we released the micro-clamps and the artery immediately flowed well. We called 'Flap on!' and Bhindhi at once worked out the ischaemic time. In Faisal's case, the flap had gone without blood and oxygen supply for forty-eight minutes. We then attached the front wall of the flap vein to Faisal's neck vein, but had to flip it over to do the rest of the vein, which can be difficult to get right because the smaller of the two veins can twist in on itself. Blood carrying tissue-nourishing oxygen was the key for the survival of Faisal's new face, but this particular reconstruction flap had no area of external skin that the nursing and medical team in Intensive Care could see, making monitoring of the success or failure of the reconstructed face very difficult. However, the Doppler microprobe we attached to the flap vein told us that blood was whooshing through the flap, allowing us to relax a little.

We finished the inset of the flap to reconstruct the tumour defect, making sure that, once his scars had healed, Faisal's face, chin and mouth, and his ability to speak, chew food and swallow, would be as good as they were before the tumour had begun to form. We also made sure that the flap was absolutely watertight all the way round, and wouldn't allow saliva to leak from the mouth into the neck, which would have led to infection.

We checked again that everything was still running well and there was no worrying signal from the Doppler microprobes, and then we started to close, placing drains in Faisal's neck to allow fluid to escape, aiding the healing process. When we closed the area from which the flap had been harvested, we carefully placed the incised edges together and sewed them in layers. There was no need for a tummy tuck on this occasion: Faisal was young and fit enough not to need any extra help in the washboard department. With the operation complete, the still sleeping Faisal was then wheeled out of the theatre and transferred to a bed in the High Dependency Unit, where he would be continuously monitored by specialist nurses and kept pain-free.

When we woke him, Faisal was not exactly looking his best. Bloody fluid from his wounds was seeping out through the drain tubes on either side of his neck. He had an arterial line in his wrist, an IV drip in his arm and a maze of other tubes and wires connecting him to the monitoring systems that were keeping him safe, their monotone beeping as reassuring a sound to the trained ear as the *whoosh* of the Doppler probe. His face and neck were marked by the long, faint line of a scar from below his right ear, crossing obliquely down and forward and then running around his neck in a skin crease. Inside his mouth there were also multiple purple 'mattress sutures', making a watertight seal to hold the graft in place. His face on the lower right side was so swollen that it looked at least twice its normal size, and the swelling would make it impossible for him to open his mouth or turn his head for some time. By the time a couple of days had passed, he would look even worse, as his bruised tissues discoloured.

His facial swelling, the bruises and the general numbness of his face would take at least a fortnight to fade, although he would be up and out of bed pretty well straight away. He would also be on a very strict liquids-only diet at first, and soft foods for even longer; it would be six weeks before he could eat his first proper solid meal. This was not the time to mention any of that to Faisal, of course, and I was confident that, by the time the healing process was complete, his face would be fully restored to its previous handsome, unmarked, youthful condition.

I stood beside his bed as his eyelids flickered open and he looked up at me through woozy, unfocused eyes.

'Everything's fine, Faisal,' I said. 'It all went really well.'

All I got in reply was a sleepy grunt from him, but that was enough.

When I phoned Faisal's parents immediately after I'd been to see him in the HDU, I could hear the relief in his father's voice as he stammered out his thanks and then relayed the gist of my message to his wife. That is always the moment when I feel overwhelmingly privileged, even when there are no other words left to say.

Faisal's operation proved to be a complete success, but even for such a fit and healthy young man his recuperation was a long, slow process and his pain from both operation sites – his rebuilt jaw and the iliac crest from which we'd taken the transplanted flap – often proved difficult to control. Unsurprisingly, there were times during the following weeks when he was very down. Nonetheless, despite his pain, the first thing he always asked me every time he hobbled through the door of my office on his crutches was, 'When will I be able to get back in the pool?' And I'd always have to say, 'Trust me, Faisal, you will, just not quite yet.'

'But when?'

'As soon as possible. But in the meantime, this is what I need you to do.' And I'd begin outlining yet another programme of rehabilitation or a course of physiotherapy for him to follow.

When he finally walked into my consulting rooms one day with a broad smile on his face, having at last discarded his crutches, there was no looking back for him. Not long afterwards he and his proud parents showed me a video of him back in the swimming pool, with a lane all to himself. It was a special session, arranged by his coach, just to get him going again and rebuild his confidence in the water. As I watched the footage on Faisal's laptop, I was very aware of his penetrating gaze fixed on me.

When I got to the end of the video, I turned to look at him and let the silence build for a few seconds before giving a slow shake of my head. 'Jesus,' I said, deadpan. 'If you'd gone any slower, Faisal, you'd have sunk!'

He stared at me for a moment, slack-jawed, and then burst out laughing. I could sense the relief washing through him, and the glow of parental pride filling the room. He's now training hard again, has grown another three inches in the last year, and is challenging for honours with his regional swimming team. He walked into my clinic recently, towering over me and his parents, his broad shoulders straining the seams of his giant-sized school blazer, and said, 'I want to have that swim race with you now!' The confident boy I'd first met was back.

3

NO SANE PERSON would dispute the value of the life-saving maxillofacial surgery we carry out to remove a cancerous tumour, or repair and rebuild the face of a victim of trauma caused by a car crash, a gunshot, an explosion, a fall or an assault. Cosmetic surgery remains a much more controversial issue, usually the so-called vanity projects sometimes funded by the NHS that the tabloid newspapers love to cover; but many of the procedures I carry out are to restore the appearance of patients who have first undergone major operations after trauma or diagnosis with cancer, and sometimes, even when no visible trace of the surgery remains and their face has healed perfectly, it's necessary to carry out further cosmetic work to restore the symmetry of their features.

One of my maxillofacial patients, for example – Geoff – was a middle-aged man who had crashed on his mountain bike and given himself a deep-plane face-lift in the process, or at least the first part of one. On admission to hospital, his wounds were full of dirt and debris that had to be debrided (cleaned out) and the wounds closed, prior to major trauma reconstruction. We used titanium plates and screws to reposition the bones around his eye and the soft tissues were then repositioned, reconstructed and reattached to restore his looks as close as possible to the way they had been before the accident. We often request a photograph from relatives to aid this process.

The operation was a complete success and, once healed, there were no visible facial scars at all, but the repositioned tissue resulted in Geoff appearing ten years younger on that side of his face than on the undamaged one. Cosmetic surgery to the other side of his face was then necessary to balance his looks, so the lasting result of his accident was to make that forty-five-year-old man look not a day over thirty-five. It's doubtful if I have ever had a more satisfied patient!

Another of my patients, a young woman called Deirdre, was a much more complex case. She had also suffered major facial trauma, in her case after being a passenger in the back seat of a car involved in a serious accident. She was thrown face-first through a side window, suggesting that she wasn't wearing a seatbelt at the time of impact. The car had rolled over several times and she had suffered horrific facial injuries. As well as the trauma from the impacts, there was a lot of glass damage to her face, something that used to be much more frequent before the laws on wearing seatbelts were introduced. The glass used in car windows is safety glass that doesn't break into jagged fragments so it doesn't lacerate the flesh to the extent that you would bleed to death, but it does break into tiny cubes, causing horrible little scars that are difficult to treat.

The facial skeleton forms a cage that protects the brain, with the spaces within the sinus, the thin sections of bone and weak joints creating a 'crumple zone' in the central part of the face that absorbs impacts and blunt force in the same way as the grilles on the front of an SUV. Deirdre's crumple zone had absorbed most of the impact of the crash, but unfortunately she had suffered an inter-cranial injury as well. Her brain was swollen, and while it was in that condition it was touch-and-go whether she would survive at all, so we obviously didn't want to expose her to any more anaesthetic or surgery than was absolutely essential until the swelling had come down again.

In time she recovered, and when she first came to see me, my colleagues at Glasgow had already pretty much reconstructed her face from scratch, so much so that a steel wire beneath the flesh held the two halves of her face together and the central strut of her nose was a bit of bone from the top of her skull. However, as a result of such severe trauma, the soft tissues of the face had scarred down to their new positions faster than we could get at them to reposition them, so the results of the initial reconstruction had not been quite right. The good news was that we could still make adjustments, and luckily her facial nerves had survived intact, so everything was moving and operating correctly.

The accident had happened when Deirdre was a young woman; she was still only twenty when she came to see me and was still in the process of recovery. As well as the physical trauma, she was also having to deal with all the psychological trauma that went with it. One of the additional problems I had to solve for her was that, having already received the settlement for her injuries from the driver's insurance company, she had then undergone an extensive series of cosmetic procedures at a private clinic, and not only to her face: she'd had buttock implants as well.

The end result of all this was much less successful than it should have been, and when I first saw Deirdre it was evident that I not only needed to complete the good work my colleagues had done in repairing the trauma damage and rebuilding the structures of her face, I also had to counter some of the effects of her subsequent, inexpert cosmetic surgery. That had left her with visible scarring on her face – and after her injuries and the initial reconstruction, the last thing she needed was more scars. She also had severe-looking, semi-permanent eyebrows that were too angular and not the right curved shape for her face, there was too much botox in her forehead, and much too much filler in her lips. She wanted more but I refused to do that because her lips already looked unnaturally swollen and in my view it was not at all an attractive look.

However, I was able to remove and adjust some of the visible scars on her face, enhancing her appearance, and there were a series of other minor improvements I made for her, including sculpting her upper lip to improve the look of her mouth, and slightly adjusting the shape of her left eye to match her right. Those changes had a big overall impact, without pumping yet more filler into her lips or doing any extreme procedures to her face.

I did use some filler, though. Deirdre had also complained that her nose was too straight, making it look artificial. She was quite right, because it was a straight piece of the outer layer of her skull that had been used to give her a new nose. Rather than carry out further surgery on that (and after all her previous operations it was such a mass of scar tissue that the blood flow through it was not good anyway, making any further operations dauntingly complex), I was able to inject a tiny amount of filler into the tip of her nose, giving it a much more natural and aesthetically pleasing look. It is remarkable how little filler you need to transform someone's face completely. The syringes we use look fairly big, because they are glass-walled and quite thick, but they never contain more than one millilitre, and often as little as 0.55ml. A teaspoon holds 5ml, so we are talking tiny amounts here, but they can have a quite disproportionate effect.

While for Geoff and Deirdre cosmetic surgery was the necessary corollary to their trauma surgery – even if in Deirdre's case it had been much overdone – part of my work is also to carry out purely cosmetic procedures on patients who have no underlying medical or surgical problems. Mary was an attractive woman in her late forties, but her face showed some of the natural signs of ageing, and in her case they had been heightened by the effects of heavy cigarette smoking over many years. The first time she came to see me, bringing a friend with her for moral support, she sat down and poured it all out to me, her eyes filling with tears as she spoke. Her only daughter was getting married in six weeks' time – something that every mother should be looking forward to – and all the family and guests were flying out to Majorca for the ceremony and a party to celebrate it, but Mary was dreading the trip because she was so depressed about the way she looked. Things had been brought to a head after a cruel comment by someone she knew (this is a common thread in many of the cases I see) and it had been the trigger for her seeking cosmetic treatment.

As usual with a new patient, I first spent time getting to know a little bit about her. She was a Yorkshire housewife and her husband, whom I met on her next visit, was a big, gruff, archetypal Yorkshire taxi driver. They were clearly not wealthy people who were throwing their money around just for the sake of it. Every major item of expenditure had to be thought through, even agonized over, so the fact that she was even contemplating spending a fairly large sum on cosmetic treatment showed how concerned she was about the way she looked and how much her confidence had been hit by that.

Her brow was drawn down into a semi-permanent frown and she had quite pronounced jowls. We never lose the tone of the muscle immediately around our mouths because it's constantly in motion when we're talking, chewing, smiling and frowning, but the fat pad under our cheeks does lose tone as we age and moves down and forward to form jowls around the mouth. The skin under her eyes wasn't too bad, but the loose skin over her eyelids had given her the 'hooded' look that many people's eyes have in later years, though in Mary's case it was so pronounced it was beginning to affect her vision. The skin was so irregular that she was even finding it difficult to apply her eye make-up because it piled up in lumps and got caught in the folds. That was further damaging her already fragile confidence, making her feel even less attractive. Like every proud mother, she wanted to be at her best on her daughter's wedding day, but though she could have her hair and her make-up done, choose a lovely outfit and all the rest of it, without cosmetic treatment she couldn't do anything about the way her eyelids looked.

I was confident that I could make a big difference to her appearance, so when she asked me, 'Can you do something about my eyelids, doctor?', I said, 'Yes I can, but I'd want to do the operation right, and get your brow in a better position as well. So I'd like to give you a chemical brow-lift – a botox injection, in other words. I'll just put a little into the muscles low down in the middle of your forehead to pull your brow back up but without giving you so much that you finish up with a brow like a billiard table, because at our age, Mary, that isn't necessarily aesthetically pleasing. There should be a tiny line there and you want your face to be expressive, not a mask. I'll also do a little bit of work on the flesh surrounding the eyes, as well as sorting out the problem with your eyelids with a small operation to get rid of the excess skin.'

My anxiety was that it was only six weeks to the wedding and I wouldn't be able to get the best possible result for her in that time. In six months we'd be getting closer to it, but she would still be improving a year later, especially if she let me keep the botox injections up, because the dermis underneath tightens and the muscles get used to the idea. So in an ideal world we would have been having the discussion a year earlier, but we were where we were and I was still confident we could make a big improvement in her looks by the time of the wedding. It would be a two-stage process: there would be a big improvement after the first treatment with botox, and a further improvement after a second dose in three to four months' time. That would be too late for the wedding, of course, but I promised her that after the minor surgery and the chemical treatment to her brow she would see a significant improvement within a few days.

'However, there is one thing that I need you to do for me first, Mary,' I added, 'and that is to stop smoking, even if it's only for the period around the operation, because even that short time without cigarettes will make a big difference, whereas carrying out the operation while you are still smoking will greatly increase the risks to you.'

Cancer and ageing have always been two sides of the same coin. Smoking fills your haemoglobin (which should be transporting oxygen) with carbon monoxide (CO) and constricts your arteries, and the haemoglobin doesn't get rid of the CO easily. It can give you a cherry red complexion – fire victims who've been inhaling smoke often look pinker than they would naturally – and those flat hydrocarbon molecules slot in between the DNA chains and cause mutations which are the principal mechanisms by which cancer develops from tobacco usage. So the CO that comes from tobacco smoke is a big part of the problem. Secondary smoking is also damaging to a person's looks as well as their health. Even if you don't smoke yourself, if you're sharing a house with a smoker, your haemoglobin will carry some of that CO, your skin will age faster and your looks will deteriorate quicker than those of a non-smoker in a non-smoking house.

Mary was giving me a sceptical look, so I told her, 'This isn't the usual "smoking causes cancer" lecture, Mary – though it does. But smoking also damages the healing process and greatly increases the chances of you picking up a post-operative infection, and with only six weeks to go to the wedding, that would be a disaster. I can treat the infection, if it occurs, and cure it with antibiotics, but it will slow down the healing process and give you a lumpy scar and eyes that look like somebody has thumped you, and that is definitely not what you want for your daughter's wedding photographs. So really, truly, do you think you could stop smoking?'

She thought for a moment. 'How long would I have to stop for?'

That was a bit of a 'how long is a piece of string' question, but you can clear the carbon monoxide from your system in forty-eight hours. If someone really can't manage without nicotine, then vaping is better than smoking because you don't get carbon monoxide from vaping devices. You do still get constriction of the blood vessels from the nicotine, though, so even with vaping, less blood is flowing around the body and that will slow healing and recovery rates, but at least when the blood is flowing it is carrying oxygen and not carbon monoxide so it won't starve the blood and fill it with toxins the way tobacco does.

I took a deep breath. 'If you can give up altogether for those few days, that will make a big improvement. And I tell you what, in just a few days without smoking, you'll notice a difference in your skin tone too.' I held her gaze. 'So, do you think you could be a non-smoker for at least a week? Then we can do this for you next Friday. Can you do that for me?'

She looked me in the eye and said, 'I'll definitely do it, doctor.'

Sure enough, when Mary returned for her pre-op consultation, she assured me – and I believed her – that she had not touched a cigarette since our first meeting and had just been vaping when she needed a cigarette. 'OK, well done,' I said, 'but if you can just tone down the vaping as well now, either side of the op, that would be really helpful because then the blood flow will be as good as we can make it.'

She managed to do that too, and when I saw her on the morning of the operation she wasn't at all nervous, just excited.

Having got her into the operating theatre, I used botox to adjust her brow muscle to the right position, reduced her jowls, tightened up the flesh around her eyes a little, and did a blepharoplasty – the excision of part of the skin of the upper eyelids. There was a lot of loose skin there but you always remove what seems like a remarkably large amount of upper eyelid tissue in a blepharoplasty anyway – you only leave seven to nine millimetres of the eyelid skin and ten of the brow skin above the lid, and all the rest is cut away. So the correct response from one of my trainees the first time they see me doing an 'upper bleph' is 'Jesus! Are you sure?' because it looks like you're taking much too much away. You take a tiny amount of the muscle with the skin as well, but that helps the muscle tighten up afterwards.

It should be the case when you've finished the operation – and it's best to do it with the patient awake – that they can't quite close their eyes. That can be very alarming for them, so I always explain the reason beforehand: the skin is going to stretch again afterwards, so that gives the best result. You also have to be very careful not to touch the gland that produces tears. I have to warn my patients that due to swelling after the operation, the eye will sometimes feel dry because the blinking mechanism that normally delivers tears doesn't work quite so well until the swelling goes down again.

Mary's operation went really well. Although, as I had warned her, the reduction of lines on the forehead is a gradual process that takes about six months to reach its full effect, botox only takes seven to ten days to work and the impact of a blepharo-plasty is almost immediate. So by the time she came back to see me just seven days later, even though she still had quite a bit of oedema (swelling), she was already looking much better, and more importantly feeling much better about herself. With every patient having that kind of procedure I always warn them that they're going to go through the mill and they're going to get some bruising – not a black eye as if they've been punched, but blood is going to track round and give them a blue and then later a yellowish discolouration like a fading bruise. Mary had had all that, but when she came in to see me that was already disappearing and she was smiling broadly.

She said that when the nurses took the stitches out before she came to see me, they told her 'You're healing really fast' and one of them had said to her, 'I've never seen a blepharoplasty heal this well, this quickly.' So she was absolutely thrilled with that. She had spent a fair bit of cash on all sorts of aspects of the wedding, as you do, but she told me that she didn't regret a penny of the money she had spent on the op. She just had one complaint: 'I keep getting the feeling that people are staring at me.'

'They probably are, Mary,' I said. 'And do you know why they're staring at you? It's because they see such an improvement in the way you look and they don't know what's happened. You haven't gone round telling people you're having surgery, have you?'

She shook her head.

'I thought not, people almost never do. So your friends and neighbours can see this dramatic improvement in you and they're just trying to work out why you look different, that's all. You look refreshed and well, so they're staring at you for all the right reasons: because you look so good.'

By the time she came back for a second review, she was wearing full make-up, including the eye make-up she'd been unable to apply before. She looked stunning, and there were no more concerns about people staring at her; she was loving it! She told me she felt – and she certainly looked – ten years younger. She was positively glowing. In fact she was so thrilled with the results of her treatment that, despite having already paid a handsome sum to the clinic, she turned up having bought cakes for all the staff and a box of shortbread for me as well. She also gave me a card that read 'Dear Professor McCaul, I am so delighted with the outcome and I am now really looking forward to my daughter's wedding.' Instead of the downcast, tearful person who had come in a few weeks earlier almost dreading the thought of attending her daughter's big day, she was now brimming with confidence and actively wanting to be in the pictures rather than hiding herself from the photographer.

Mary encapsulated for me the joy of performing what is a relatively minor operation but one that has to be carried out absolutely meticulously in order to produce the right result. She wasn't someone wanting some daft or extreme treatment so she could look like a Hollywood movie star or the latest Instagram sensation, she was just a nice, normal person who wanted to look a little bit better for her age. So show me someone who says we shouldn't be carrying out those kinds of cosmetic procedures and I'll introduce them to Mary and they can try to convince her.

Botox therapy has been in use for over thirty years and is an extremely safe and proven procedure; the number of disasters and deaths associated with it is zero. So in the right medical hands it's a perfectly reasonable thing to have done. Critics inevitably focus on cases where it's overdone, like young women having too much filler inserted in their lips, or older people in the public eye who effectively 'binge' on botox or other cosmetic procedures (and I'm sure we can all think of A-, B- and C-list celebrities to whom this applies). Some have even employed their own nurses and extra measures to get around the regulation that botox has to be prescribed by a medically qualified person. In that situation, it seems they are able to access as many botox injections as they feel like and, like those who have undergone facial plastic surgery too frequently for far too long, they can end up looking terrible.

I would never allow a patient of mine to go to those extremes, but sensible cosmetic procedures are perfectly acceptable. A lot of people may feel that this area of medical treatment is all about personal vanity, but while that may be true in some cases, most of the work I do in that area, just like Mary's surgery, is really about personal dignity, not vanity.

As we grow older, all of us show the signs of ageing to a greater or lesser extent. Since we spend the majority of our lives upright, the force of gravity makes some elements of the face descend, so facial volume shifts, generally being lost from the top of the face and accumulating at the bottom, hollowing out the temples and heading south. Lines and folds form on our skin, facial tissues droop, forming bags beneath the eyes and jowls around our mouths, our eyelids can become hooded and our skin loses its elasticity. Our noses and ears also get larger as we age because, albeit slowly, cartilage continues to grow throughout our lives. Most of these changes can be addressed surgically and non-surgically and they tend to be the things that people want to improve. The aim is – or should be – to fix things in a way that is not harmful, so the patient just looks a little bit better: good for their age rather than ridiculously youthful.

If our surgical team can enhance the quality of life for an individual, whether it's a patient recovering from cancer, someone wanting to keep their job, or even if it's just that they're ageing and would like to look better, why would we not do it? The most important thing in the field of cosmetic treatment (defined as a procedure for someone with no pathology other than ageing changes) is to manage expectations. First, get to know the patient, then decide if what they want is deliverable and make sure they understand the potential outcomes and limitations of what can be done before going ahead. Don't jump straight in with an operation, as some clinics do, undertaking treatments for financial reasons on patients who may not be psychologically stable enough to have them. Unfortunately a small number of people do have psychological problems that no amount of cosmetic surgery will fix. Some have a psychological/pathological condition called body dysmorphia, meaning that they feel there is something wrong with their body shape, and most often their face, and no amount of cosmetic enhancement will convince them otherwise. It's very important to identify people with that condition at once, because no matter what you do they won't be satisfied with it. Other forms of help are more appropriate.

Whether I agree to operate on someone depends on many factors, all carefully assessed at more than one meeting. Apart from assessment of ageing changes in the face, an important early consideration is their reasons for wanting to have treatment at this particular point in time. My assessment of whether surgical or non-surgical treatment will improve their looks and their quality of life is secondary to this. So the opening of my consultations always covers the same ground: not only 'How can I help?' but also 'Why have you decided to do something about it now?' If the response is not reasonable (an extreme example could be 'My husband's just left me and I want him to come back'), intervention is contra-indicated. While feeling desperately sorry for someone in such a position, this is a bad reason for seeking treatment: it is unlikely to lead to a good outcome overall for that person and adding surgery to difficult life events is not appropriate. As a senior surgeon years ago said to me, 'If all marital problems could be solved by cosmetic surgery, there'd be far fewer divorces.'

The next question covers their medical history – general details about past and current illnesses and medicines, and then 'What treatments have you had in the past?' We also need to establish if patients have any allergies to medicines or dressings and, importantly, if they have ever been in hospital for any illnesses or operations. Those questions will establish everything we need to know about the medical side of things.

Then comes the question 'Who do you live with at home and what work do you do?' In terms of cosmetic treatment, the latter is often germane. I've treated everyone from average men and women to television presenters – male and female – and if someone is in the public eye, whether on the TV or as a receptionist on a company's front desk, there is pressure, sometimes overt, sometimes less so, to look their best, and they can feel that their jobs are under threat if they don't 'look right'.

The key question is 'Do you smoke or drink alcohol?' Excessive alcohol consumption damages your looks as well as your health, but there is no doubt that, quite apart from the cancer risks, tobacco use is the most deleterious activity in terms of facial ageing. It's a message we should get out more because one of the strange paradoxes of my work is that there is a tendency for patients to make light of health warnings about the effect of smoking on cancer risk and heart disease. That makes it a hard sell when 'all' I'm going to be doing is performing potentially life-saving surgery to remove a tumour, but if I tell my patients that smoking is threatening their looks, they're much more likely to take the warning seriously and do something about it.

4

THE FIRST TIME I can clearly remember wanting to be a surgeon was when I was just seven years old. I'd seen some medical dramas like *General Hospital* on the tiny black and white TV in our cramped living room, but from a very early age I'd also been aware of my polio-stricken mother's constant pain. She had contracted the disease when she was two, soon after her baby brother was born. The family doctor dismissed it at first as 'attention-seeking behaviour', fuelled by jealousy of the fuss being made of the new baby. But when she then developed a high fever and started to walk with an awkward, halting gait, throwing her right leg out to the side with each step, the paralysis of her muscles was finally recognized and diagnosed.

My mother spent many months in hospital over the course of the next few years and had surgery at the Royal Hospital for Sick Children in Glasgow on three separate occasions. She can still vividly recall the isolation she and many other children had to endure after undergoing major surgery in that 'children should be seen and not heard' era. There was rarely, if ever, any attempt to explain to her or to her parents what had been done, or was about to be done, to her, nor when she could expect to recover and be out of hospital, just endless long and lonely days with no company, very few distractions, and only the all-too-brief visits by her parents during evening visiting time – strictly limited to one hour – to look forward to.

Children were not allowed to visit at all, and she has a haunting memory of her younger brother having to wait outside while their parents were with her. He pressed his palms against the outside of the window of her ground-floor ward while she held hers against the inside, so that their hands were almost touching, and both of them were in tears at their enforced separation. She also remembers waking up after yet another operation and making the traumatic, panic-stricken discovery of a blood-filled plaster cast on her leg and a spreading crimson stain on those crisp white hospital sheets, and having to be rushed back into the operating theatre for yet more surgery.

When she was eventually discharged from hospital she was given callipers to support her damaged leg but found the weight of them very difficult, quite apart from the stigma of having to wear them at a time when large sections of British society still appeared to equate physical disability with a corresponding lack of intellectual ability. It took her several years to recover from her missed schooling, but despite having to start in the lowest stream in her first year at secondary school she had risen to the A-stream by the time she reached the fourth form.

She was advised to have further surgery in her teens but refused it so that she could sit her Lowers and Highers (then the Scottish equivalent of GCSEs and A Levels). She duly passed them all, but even then, before she was accepted for a teacher training course she still had to convince the nuns at Notre Dâme College in Glasgow that the fact that she had a polio-damaged leg did not mean she was mentally deficient as well. Her tenacity and perseverance eventually saw her overcome all the obstacles put in her way, and she successfully completed her training and became a primary school teacher, just as she had always dreamed.

Her polio had first been diagnosed in 1948, just after the launch of the National Health Service, and I have often reflected that had the NHS not been created, providing treatment for all, regardless of their ability to pay, my mum's parents might not have been able to afford her life-changing surgery. Before the NHS was founded there was a rudimentary National Insurance Scheme for those in work, but the modest benefits were paid only to contributors, not their dependants; they were paid at a flat rate regardless of the severity of the illness, and they only covered limited care by a doctor. Contributors were only entitled to hospital treatment if they were suffering from tuberculosis, which had reached plague proportions in Britain (over 46,000 British people died of it in the peak year of 1918, and around 20,000 people a year were still dying of it in the 1940s). All other conditions requiring hospitalization had to be paid for at the full market rate. If a birth led to medical complications, that too had to be paid for.

As a result of the restrictions, low-income families had invariably struggled to find the money to pay the fee for a visit to the doctor, let alone an operation, and often resorted to quack remedies, or simply hoped that an ill family member would get better by themselves. Sometimes they did, but sometimes curable conditions were left untreated until too late, with damaging or even fatal consequences.

When the NHS was set up by the Minister of Health Aneurin Bevan on 5 July 1948, it was based on three founding principles: that it meet the needs of everyone; that it be free at the point of delivery; and that it be based on clinical need, not ability to pay. Seventy years later, despite the ever-louder right-wing sniping from the sidelines, those founding principles remain at the heart of the National Health Service.

Without the advent of the NHS, my mother might never have been able to become a teacher and might never have met my dad, so the direct impact of the NHS on my family is tangible. The care she received allowed our family to go on to produce a professor of maxillofacial surgery (me) and also a consultant paediatric orthopaedic surgeon – my baby sister Janet, who has recently been appointed a consultant surgeon in the very same department in the very same hospital where our mother was treated all those years ago. So it is very clear to me that, despite its faults, the NHS continues to be the most prized possession of us all. It delights me that our family is contributing to it so directly, and the attempts by ideologues to denigrate it, weaken it or even abolish it altogether leave me horrified and furious.

When I was growing up, the presence of polio in our home was daily emphasized by the aching and burning pain my mum suffered in her leg, particularly in her knee. She tried not to let it show, but as she moved around the kitchen I'd often see her wince and bite her lip. At the end of a particularly uncomfortable day she'd sit in front of the old electric fire in the kitchen, her foot resting on the low wooden steps she used when getting things down from the top shelves in the larder, and my brother and I would take it in turns to massage her knee, keeping it up until our hands were aching. There was no other palliative treatment available; her pain was just 'the cross she had to bear', as people used to say back then. Only very recently, as my mother's generation has aged with the aftermath of the disease, has a post-polio pain syndrome at last been properly recognized and treatments devised to try to alleviate it.

Looking back now on my seven-year-old self, I suppose I must have been vaguely aware that the medical profession was held in high regard and that it was an honourable, respected career, but there was certainly no thought in my mind of that, nor of earning a high income or anything like that. I just remember thinking that if I learned how to be a surgeon, I'd be able to make my mother's pain go away.

Medicine wasn't the most obvious career for the son of a relatively low-income family living in a rented house in a working-class district of Glasgow. When my parents were first married they lived in Linwood, a few miles south-west of the city, because being a primary school teacher there gave my mum the right to a council house. There was a huge car factory at Linwood, and it was a thriving community, but when the factory was closed down in 1981, with the remaining production transferred to the West Midlands, people began to leave in droves. There was virtually no alternative work in the area and the town went downhill fast. Two of the local primary schools eventually closed for lack of pupils and the whole place assumed a growing air of dereliction. The once-neat estate where we had lived was scarred by abandoned houses with rubbish, broken furniture and rotting mattresses dumped among the weeds in their overgrown gardens. Shops were boarded up, walls and shutters were sprayed with graffiti, and junkies' needles glinted among the broken glass and litter in the dark corners of the crumbling concrete walkways. It was no longer somewhere you would choose to walk alone at night, nor to live if you had the funds to move elsewhere.

When he left school, my dad had joined one of the great Glasgow marine engineering firms, first as an engineering apprentice and later as a draughtsman, before finally becoming a contract engineer. He and my mum worked hard and saved even harder, and eventually they managed to put together the money for a mortgage, whereupon we moved, first to a house on a 1970s new-build estate, and later to a detached house in the leafy suburb of Bishopton. There were no 'Streets' in Bishopton. Every thoroughfare was, at the least, a 'Road', and usually a 'Crescent', 'Grove' or 'Avenue'. That only served to reinforce Bishopton's posh image at my secondary school in Renfrew, where anyone who came from there tended to be labelled 'a snob'. If you were also reasonably bright you were doubly suspect, and your sexuality was challenged as well. It was certainly character forming; you either sank or swam.

Another red rag to the school bullies was that I was learning to play the flute. Much as I now hate to admit it, it was listening to James Galway on the radio in our home in Bishopton when I was a kid that had first interested me in the instrument and my choice of it was simply because I loved the sound he made. I was seven at the time and already playing the recorder after my brother and I had both been given one the previous Christmas. I was desperate to have a crack at the flute as well, but there was no music tuition at my primary school and it wasn't until I was at secondary school that I had a chance to try it, so I started relatively late, aged eleven, and even then it needed all of my mother's legendary persistence to get me some lessons.

Mum was only four feet eleven-and-a-half inches tall but she was a very feisty character; as she always used to say, 'The best things come in small packages . . . but then so does poison!' She had dark curly hair and was very beautiful – she was the Gala Day Queen at the Rolls-Royce factory when my grandpa used to work there – but she was also fiercely intelligent and a very motivated woman who could have given captains of industry seminars on assertiveness. When something didn't suit her, although she would just very politely say 'No, thank you', you could almost hear the clasp of her handbag snapping shut, to leave you in no doubt that once her mind was made up, no amount of counter-argument was going to alter it.

So when she phoned the Head of Music for the whole Strathclyde region to ask if he could arrange for me to have flute lessons, she wasn't going to take 'No' for an answer. Despite her persistence, he made no promises to her during their conversation, but he then suffered a heart attack shortly afterwards and was off work for some time. This was very unfortunate for him but very lucky for me because, seizing her chance, my mum immediately phoned up his replacement and, with her fingers firmly crossed behind her back, said, 'The Head of Music promised that he'd arrange for my son to have some flute lessons.' He believed her and arranged it.

My brother Vincent had meanwhile opted to learn the trumpet. In retrospect he may have come to see that as something of a mistake, because he was forced to practise it in what my dad described as 'the acoustic enclosure', better known to the rest of us as the cupboard under the stairs. My dad also insisted that he keep the door shut while he was in there, muting the volume for the rest of us but practically deafening my poor brother inside. Despite the enclosed practice environment, Vincent thrived, eventually gravitating to jazz rather than classical music.

Since the flute was a relatively quiet and tuneful instrument, unlike my brother I was allowed to practise in the wide open spaces of the dining room, under the watchful eye of my grandparents and great-grandparents, frozen forever in our array of family photographs wearing the half-proud, half-fearful expression their generation always seemed to adopt when facing a camera.

The music teacher I had been assigned was sufficiently impressed with the results of my basic flute lessons to take me to see a specialist tutor in the instrument, a flautist called Sheena, who played in the Scottish Chamber Orchestra. She earned extra money by giving advanced flute lessons, and after I auditioned for her, she took me on as a pupil. Like my mum she was just under five feet tall, with short dark hair and a ready smile, and like my mum she was dynamic, focused, and completely inspirational. She had a different way of thinking about things and was very supportive, but she did not suffer fools. If you turned up for a lesson without having practised, watch out! I did so once, partly because I didn't much like the piece we were playing that week, and after a couple of minutes she held up her hand to stop me, gave me a hard stare and said, 'Don't ever turn up that badly prepared again.' I really took that to heart and from then on I always practised hard.

After Sheena had satisfied herself that I really was willing to work to make myself a better player, she gave me one of the flute head joints (the part nearest the mouth) that she owned, a beautiful silver one, inlaid with gold – I still have it – and the sound it made was fabulous. It transformed my playing, and having joined the Royal Scottish Academy of Music and Drama, I used it all the way through my time with them and in performances with the junior orchestras I also joined.

I had been picked for the school football team as well but I had to give that up because flute lessons and playing in the orchestra took up every Saturday. Stopping football did not go down well with my schoolmates, but I absolutely loved my music. My dad was very supportive of my choice, and would often say, 'You can play music your whole life, but you can't play football for the whole of it' – though, come to think of it, that might have invited the retort 'So I should make the most of football while I can, then?'

As I developed as a flautist, I soon discovered that there was a lot of quiet, deep satisfaction in practising something and feeling it slowly but steadily getting better. In flute playing, as in other areas of life, you reach a tipping point where, after thinking 'I can't do it, I just can't do it', all of a sudden you can. Learning the flute was the first time in my life that I mastered something complex. The finger movements were technically difficult but flute playing requires much more than just manual dexterity: it's the whole combination of breathing, relaxation and posture, along with the technical skill to play the instrument.

The best way I found to succeed was to repeat and repeat and repeat. If I found a piece difficult, I set myself to do it ten times, and if I made a mistake on the ninth recital I had to do another ten. However, as well as repetitions, it could also be about distraction. Sheena would sometimes say, 'Right, I want you to really focus on your right big toe while you play it again.' It sounds mad, but suddenly the right side of your brain, if you're right-handed, has achieved what you wanted, because the left side of your brain that kept thinking 'I can't do it, I just can't do it' – the anxious brain if you like – has been silenced by being forced to focus on something else, allowing the part that is innate to take over. This technique comes from the 'Inner Game' school. First used about golf and then tennis, the term was also employed to describe the technical challenges of high-level musical performance. So that's how you do it in music, and there is a direct parallel between playing technically difficult flute passages and surgical skill, because it can also be how you do it in microsurgery, when you're staring down the microscope and something seems unfeasibly difficult. It's a similar principle, the way one will focus, concentrate, and then relax and get something to happen – but with completely different stakes, of course.

I eventually became a good enough musician to play first flute in the orchestra at the Royal Scottish Academy of Music and Drama, and for a while I even had vague thoughts of becoming a professional, but then, as now, the employment prospects for musicians were not bright and Sheena told me very firmly, 'If there is anything else you can do to earn a good living, you should do that instead and just enjoy your music without trying to make a living from it.'

That was enough to convince me to pursue my original interest in Medicine. But whether distracted by music, or more likely by my discovery that the opposite sex was a whole lot more interesting than I'd thought when I was younger, I ended up with grades in my fifth year that were nowhere near good enough to get me into medical school. It was a real wake-up call and I made a big effort the following year, my sixth year at senior school. I did Maths, Chemistry and Biology and managed to get an A grade in Chemistry (my Chemistry teacher excitedly told me it was the first one in the school's history) even though it was the one subject I wasn't that excited about; it just happened that I could do it well. I did OK in Maths too, because all you had to do was learn the rules, but I excelled in Biology because I had an absolute passion for it, particularly human and animal biology. It just seemed to go into a different compartment of my brain and I almost never had to be told something more than once, because I just got it straight away. Human Anatomy was like that for me, and it seemed to go hand in glove with an appreciation of classical sculpture, in which you see the anatomy beautifully defined and displayed. I used to spend hours gazing at the paintings and sculptures in the Kelvingrove Museum and Art Gallery, the Burrell Collection and the city's other museums and galleries – all of which were then free.

In the end my exam grades were two As and a B which, though a huge improvement on my results the previous year, made it touch-and-go whether I'd be able to go to medical school, where, then as now, three As was the standard requirement. However, my grades were definitely good enough to get me into dental school. That left me with a tricky decision because in those days, whether it was actually the case or not, it was widely believed that if you put a medical school as your first choice, dental schools would not offer you a place, and vice versa, so I felt I had to opt for one or the other. So after much thought, applying to dental school seemed the wiser choice.

Although I was soon doing well on my dental course and acquiring all the skills needed to become a practising dental surgeon, there was one slight problem: I had no ambition or desire to become a dental surgeon. Instead the most medical parts of the course were my principal interest. While doing some background reading about facial injuries and fractures one day, I came across some pictures of patients with facial trauma. The text alongside the images read 'These will be treated by a maxillofacial surgeon, a professional who is always doubly qualified in medicine and dentistry.' When I read that,

I thought, 'Fantastic! That's the one for me!' It was quite a eureka moment. My dental training had originally seemed a bit of a poor substitute for Medicine, but now it appeared to be the perfect first step towards my chosen vocation.

I went and had a discussion with the medical admissions tutor with a view to switching to Medicine. He asked me which speciality I wanted to practise if all went well and I answered, 'Maxillofacial surgery, for sure.'

'Well, if you're set on that speciality and you switch across to Medicine,' he said, 'you'll have to make your way in other specialities, whereas things seem to be going very well for you in Dentistry at the moment, so my advice would be to stay where you are, complete your course and then transfer to Medicine after that, if your heart is still set on becoming a maxillofacial surgeon.'

That was the best advice I could have had. He convinced me that becoming a maxillofacial surgeon was not a daft pipe-dream but that the best way into that speciality would be to complete my dental degree first. If I'd switched courses then, I'd have come out with a medical degree, but probably not a top one, whereas by staying where I was, I qualified as a Bachelor of Dental Surgery with Honours – only the third honours degree awarded by the dental school in thirty years. That was the vital first step towards my career as a maxillofacial surgeon.

My interest in maxillofacial (head and neck) surgery was reinforced by my discovery of the work of the man who was to become one of my surgical 'heroes'. Harold Delf Gillies was a New Zealand-born surgeon and pioneer of facial reconstruction. A bold experimenter and improviser, he is widely regarded as 'the father of plastic surgery'. Gillies was originally an ENT (Ear, Nose and Throat) surgeon, and only later became a maxillofacial surgeon – a speciality that had barely existed before his time, confined largely to the repair of cleft lips and palates, and fractures and deformations of the jaw. That was partly because bullets fired from the relatively crude smooth-bored rifles and handguns used until the latter part of the nineteenth century had a much lower velocity than more modern weapons and did not produce the kind of facial trauma that required major rebuilding. In addition, most such casualties occurred in overseas conflicts, and the low survival rates of wounded soldiers – because of slow transport from the battlefield, the lack of knowledge among army medics about the importance of maintaining blood volumes, and, with no antibiotics, the high death toll caused by sepsis and secondary infections – meant that few men with serious head injuries survived anyway.

I read voraciously about Gillies and his work on disfigured soldiers, poring over documents and musty-smelling books with grainy black and white illustrations, and immersing myself in his world. Gillies had grown up in Dunedin, on New Zealand's South Island. Even as a child he had a restless, enquiring mind, a sharp wit and a sometimes bizarre sense of humour. He was also an obsessive wood-carver when he was young, and the patience and meticulous attention to detail that his carving required were traits that would serve him well in his future career.

He came to England in 1903 to study natural sciences at Caius College, Cambridge, then went to the Medical College at St Bartholomew's Hospital in London (Barts for short) and was elected a Fellow of the Royal College of Surgeons in 1910. His precocious talent as a surgeon was recognized when he became assistant surgeon to Sir Milsom Rees at the ENT department of the Prince of Wales Hospital in Tottenham, whose patients included George V and many leading society figures such as Dame Nellie Melba and Alfred de Rothschild.

After the outbreak of war, Gillies enlisted in the Royal Army Medical Corps and was posted to a base hospital at Wimereux in northern France. As an anachronistic legacy of the RAMC's days as a mounted unit with horse-drawn ambulances, Gillies and the other RAMC medics were still issued with a uniform of riding breeches, field boots and spurs. In the early days of the war they even went off to tend the wounded on horseback, with their orderlies running alongside, holding on to one of the stirrups.

When Gillies landed at Boulogne, he encountered the renowned French dentist Charles Auguste Valadier, who was also on his way to Wimereux to continue his experiments with skin grafting and flap techniques to repair shrapnel wounds to men's jaws. After discussing his techniques, Valadier invited Gillies to assist him with the first operation he performed at Wimereux. Gillies also heard reports of a German surgeon, August Lindemann, who was said to be performing miracles in patching up wounded German soldiers so that they could return to the fighting, and although they were on opposite sides, Gillies did what he could to learn more about the techniques Lindemann was using.

Most of Gillies' colleagues at Wimereux returned to Britain when on leave but, inspired by what he had seen when working with Valadier, Gillies used his leave in the early summer of 1915 to travel to Paris, where he met the renowned surgeon

Hippolyte Morestin, who was also experimenting with skin flaps at the Val-de-Grâce Hospital. Morestin showed him the techniques he had developed in plastic surgery and allowed him to assist in an operation to remove a patient's facial tumour and fashion a crude repair to the defect.

Gillies later remarked that the experience 'so thrilled me that I fell in love there and then' (with facial reconstruction, not Morestin). However, while he was impressed with the Frenchman's skills, Gillies was shocked that such scant attention was paid by both Morestin and Valadier to the cosmetic effects of facial wounds. Wounded men were patched up enough to be able to go back and fight in the front lines again, but little or no attempt was made to restore their appearance and they were often left with hideous disfigurements.

Gillies returned to his RAMC unit at Wimereux determined to persuade his superiors to set up a specialist facial injuries unit, convinced that it would allow him to refine and build upon the basic techniques he had witnessed. Such were his powers of persuasion that by the end of 1915 he had been recalled to the UK to establish a facial injuries unit at the Cambridge Military Hospital, Aldershot. It had been built in 1879 to a specification suggested by Florence Nightingale, with a central corridor and wings radiating outwards, allowing in sunlight and a good circulation of air to reduce the risk of cross-infection.

Gillies had only his ENT expertise and his brief experience with Valadier and Morestin to guide him, and he had to overcome the prejudices many other surgeons held towards plastic surgery. The speciality has a history that can be traced all the way back to ancient Rome but there was little contemporary experience on which Gillies could draw, and to his surprise he learned much more from ancient texts than from modern documents. Indeed, he was startled to discover that more modern techniques were almost invariably unsuccessful unless they were based on the principles established by the classical surgeons and early nineteenth-century pioneers. 'There is hardly an operation,' Gillies remarked, 'hardly a single flap in use today that has not been suggested a hundred years ago.'

He established the new facial injuries unit with remarkable speed, and successfully performed the first operation there in February 1916. He learned by trial and error, building on his successes and learning the lessons of his agonizing failures, and was eventually able to formulate a series of 'principles' – surgical techniques – that when correctly applied would produce successful results in most cases. Although other surgeons had experimented with artificial materials, all Gillies' techniques were based on the use of living tissue taken from his patients. 'There is no royal road to the fashioning of the facial scaffold by artificial means,' he said. 'The surgeon must tread the hard and narrow way of pure surgery.' He was also relentless in his pursuit of solutions. As a ward sister at the Cambridge Military Hospital remarked, 'There was no such word as "impossible" in his vocabulary. He would not admit defeat.'

I was fascinated by the similarities and the differences between what Gillies did a century ago and the way we work today. I discovered that he had pioneered the practice of taking flaps of tissue from less visible areas of the body, usually the leg, forearm or abdomen, and using them to reconstruct the faces of soldiers disfigured by blast injuries, shrapnel or bullet wounds. Furthermore, when he began rebuilding those men's faces, he not only devised the techniques but also – because the 'tool kit' for the delicate precision work he was attempting simply didn't exist then – had to design many of his own instruments as well.

Some of these, for example, the Gillies tooth forceps – like tweezers but with a 'rat tooth' at the end, so it pinches the tissue and doesn't crush it – are still in use today and are employed for all the deep structures. If you're working on the surface, you tend to use Adsons forceps because they're a little finer, but when working deeper, the Gillies forceps, well handled, are the perfect ones for the job. The Gillies needle holders, which have a needle at the end and scissor blades higher up so you can work without an assistant and cut your own stitches, are also still in use, though I tend to prefer the ones designed by Gillies' nephew Archibald McIndoe.

Gillies' surgical techniques were just as revolutionary as the instruments he designed. For example, most cheekbone fractures are 'down and in', with the force of the impact pushing downwards and inwards towards the mouth. The traditional treatment for such fractures – operating from inside the mouth or nose – often led to infections that were very difficult to treat, so instead Gillies devised a technique of making an incision high on the temple, within the hairline. He painted the skin with iodine to prevent infection and then passed his elevator instrument (a stainless steel tool about twelve inches long, like a modified tyre iron) under the temporalis fascia (the tissue beneath the skin) but on top of the temporalis muscle (the broad, fan-shaped muscle on either side of the head). He could then click the fractured cheekbone back up and out, without the need for any incisions in the mouth or nose at all. In an era without antibiotics this was absolutely crucial because it meant that bacteria would not infect the wound. We still do it the same way today.

Gillies also found imaginative solutions to many other challenges. The difficulty of ensuring adequate blood flow to, and drainage from, transplanted flaps of tissue meant that as many as 80 per cent of transplants failed. His remarkable solution was to use 'tubed pedicles', a technique directly inspired by the sixteenth-century Italian surgeon Gaspare Tagliacozzi, which Gillies first used on William Vicarage, an Able Seaman aboard HMS *Malaya* who had been horrifically burned in a cordite explosion at the Battle of Jutland in May 1916. The explosion destroyed the soft tissues of Vicarage's ears, eyelids, nose, lips and neck, and his hands were also so badly burned that they contracted into claw-like appendages. While raising two large skin flaps from Vicarage's chest, Gillies noted their tendency to curl inwards, and had the inspiration to roll them into a tube, so that the living tissue inside it was shielded from infection by the skin on the outside.

Using this technique, he could leave one end of a skin flap attached to the donor site, ensuring a good blood supply to it, roll the flap into a tube, and then twist around the other end and attach it further up the body. He then waited until it had 'taken' in its new location, with a blood supply flowing through it, before separating the end attached to the original donor site and repeating the process. In order to replace missing facial tissue with a flap taken from the abdomen or leg, this might involve 'walking' the tissue flap up the body in a series of steps, like a caterpillar inching along a plant stem, waiting each time until viable blood flow and drainage had been established at the new site before repeating the process.

This could take weeks, or even months, so to speed things up, if the donor site was the forearm, Gillies sometimes immobilized the shoulder and elbow in a plaster cast that kept the bent forearm close to the patient's face and then attached the flap directly to its destination site. Once he was satisfied that the flap had an established blood supply in its new location, he could detach the other end from the patient's arm, though a further operation was then often necessary to straighten the arm again. While such techniques might seem crude to modern eyes, they were the only ones available at the time, and they brought about a dramatic increase in the number of successfully transplanted tissue flaps, while also helping to repair the psychological damage caused by disfigurement. With faces rebuilt, his patients could face the world with renewed confidence.

Gillies was responsible for several other great innovations and also had remarkable success with patients whom other surgeons would have written off as too disfigured to treat. They sometimes required as many as a dozen operations over the course of several years, but the results were often astonishing. For example, Lieutenant William Spreckley's nose had been completely blown off but, developing a technique described in an ancient Sanskrit text for a nose reconstruction using a flap of flesh from the forehead, Gillies created a new one for him. He implanted a piece of rib cartilage in his forehead and then, once a viable blood supply had been established, twisted it around and down, shaping it to form the new nose. The operation was a tremendous success, so much so that in later years it was difficult even to detect any scars at all on Spreckley's face. However, Gillies did note that earlier in the procedure people kept whispering behind his back about the 'elephant's trunk' he'd installed in Spreckley's forehead. Again, the technique is still used today. I did two forehead flaps in much the same way in the couple of weeks before writing this.

Gillies was far from alone in pioneering developments in his field. He assembled a cadre of elite surgeons, specialists and highly skilled nursing staff to support him, but his most significant collaborator was William Kelsey Fry,* who was doubly qualified in Dentistry and Medicine. He served as a Medical Officer in the early stages of the war but was wounded twice and invalided back to England. He was posted to the Cambridge Military Hospital, where he encountered Harold Gillies, and the two men began a collaboration that was to continue for over forty years, with Fry in charge of repairing and replacing the wounded men's broken teeth and jawbones and Gillies rebuilding their faces; or, as Fry famously remarked to him, 'I'll take the hard tissues and you take the soft.'

Fry held that every dental surgeon should be first and foremost a clinician, and only secondarily a technician, and he was a great believer in patience and a full exploration of the case history before deciding on a course of action. His famous dictum to his students was: 'God gave you ears, eyes and hands; use them on the patient in that order.'

The Cambridge Military Hospital soon proved inadequate to deal with the numbers of disfigured soldiers being sent back from the Western Front and at the end of 1916 Gillies began preparing to transfer operations to a new, much larger, dedicated unit, a 'hutted hospital' in the grounds of Frognal House

* *British Journal of Surgery*, Vol. 53, No. 4, 1966, 317-20.

in Kent. Named The Queen's Hospital, it was later renamed Queen Mary's Hospital at the insistence of the Queen, as tireless a promoter of the royal 'brand' as her husband, in return for her patronage. It was laid out in a horseshoe shape, with a central core of operating theatres and X-ray, photography and physiotherapy departments, surrounded by fourteen radiating wings, each housing beds for up to twenty-six patients.

The aim was to cater to all the British Empire wounded and it was eventually divided into four sections – British, Australian, New Zealand and Canadian – each with its own staff, mainly from those countries. American surgeons and dental surgeons also arrived after the belated entry of the United States into the war in April 1917.

The initial capacity of 320 beds was rapidly expanded to 600, and a number of outlying hospitals provided several hundred more. In order to achieve a complete cure, Gillies' patients often required multiple operations with periods of recuperation in between, and a number of other under-used hospitals and wards were requisitioned where these patients could be 'parked' to recover between the stages of the procedures to restore their faces.

To ensure he had a steady stream of mutilated soldiers to treat, Gillies had bought a load of luggage labels printed with 'Please send to Queen Mary's Hospital, Sidcup', and distributed them to nurses going to the Western Front so that they could tag soldiers with severe facial trauma and direct them to him. He expected that a total of perhaps 200 patients would arrive as a result of issuing the labels, but instead was almost overwhelmed when he found himself having to deal with ten times that number of wounded men within ten days of the new unit opening, many of them arriving still caked with mud from the battlefields. Gillies and his staff worked round the clock to deal with this avalanche of wounded men, debriding, stabilizing and dressing their wounds. The risk of secondary infections meant that all the patients' wounds had to be given daily deep cleaning using powerful disinfectants and saline solutions.

Gillies and his colleagues went on to carry out over 11,000 operations on some 5,000 patients. Many men with facial wounds were unable to eat, some were blind, deaf or incapable of speech, and most were suffering from shock, quite apart from the psychological trauma of knowing how badly disfigured they were. The French called such men *les hommes sans visages* ('the men without faces') or *les gueules cassées* ('the broken mouths'). Many of them were also suffering from depression, only too well aware of the revulsion the sight of their ravaged faces engendered, and many simply refused to return home in that condition, unwilling to allow their wives, parents or children to see them. As one of the nurses in Gillies' unit remarked, 'Hardest of all was the task of trying to rekindle the desire to live in men condemned to live week after week smothered in bandages, unable to talk, unable to taste, unable even to sleep, and all the while knowing themselves to be appallingly disfigured.'* Some men proved beyond reach and, finding their situation unendurable, committed suicide.

Gillies was well aware of the need to counter his patients' psychological trauma as well as their physical wounds. He banned mirrors from the wards and encouraged the nurses

* From H. Gillies and R. Millard, *The Principles and Art of Plastic Surgery* (Butterworth, London, 1957).

treating his patients to banter and flirt with them, giving them indirect reassurance that their personalities and attractiveness had not been obliterated by their disfigurement. He even adopted a live-wire joking, prank-playing alter ego, 'Dr Scroggie', to alleviate his patients' despair . . . and perhaps also his own. I've often used humour myself when discussing treatments and potential outcomes with my patients. It has to be sensitively judged, of course, but it is amazing how even the most feeble joke can sometimes break a sombre mood and lift a patient's spirits.

In December 1917 Gillies delivered a paper to the Medical Society of London that summed up his view of his duty as a surgeon to his adopted country in wartime. It was his responsibility, he said, firstly to 'send back to duty as many soldiers as possible in the shortest time'. His second responsibility was to the patients, to rebuild the tissue and bone that had been lost to bullet, bomb and shrapnel, but also to restore those patients' morale and self-respect. The third duty was to 'the science and knowledge of surgery'. He added that meeting all those three responsibilities simultaneously was the most difficult problem he faced.

As part of the commemoration of the centenary of the Battle of the Somme in 2016, young men dressed in First World War uniforms walked around city centres and handed out to members of the public postcards inscribed with the names of the fallen. I was given one, and for me it was a stunning and dramatic illustration of the reality not only of the numbers who died but also of their extreme youth. It made the initiative and enterprise of Harold Gillies in setting up those specialist facial injury services for young men whose visible personas had been mangled by blast, shrapnel and bullet feel even more poignant.

A typical case, showing the extent of the problems Gillies had to deal with and the multiple operations that were usually necessary, often over a period of several years, was that of Norfolk soldier Harold Page.* A butcher by trade, Page had enlisted in the army at the age of twenty-one. After nine months' basic training he was posted to France, and on 1 July 1916, the opening day of the Battle of the Somme, he was hit by a rifle or machine-gun bullet which blew off almost the whole of the right-hand side of his face. The downward trajectory of the bullet, impacting near the bridge of his nose and exiting just above the lower jaw on the right side of his face, suggests that Page was crouching, crawling on his hands and knees, or falling forward when the bullet struck him. He was blinded in his right eye and the motor- and sensory-nerve damage caused 'facial drooping' to that side of his face, as if he had suffered a stroke.

Despite the severity of his wound, Page would almost certainly have had to leave the battlefield as one of the 'walking wounded', since stretchers were used only for those incapable of making their own way back from the front lines. Wounded men were passed back through a chain of aid posts, dressing stations and casualty clearing stations to a Base Hospital like Wimereux, where Harold Gillies had worked in the early stages of the war.

* Details of Harold Page's treatment from The Gillies British Patient File of Private Harold Page, MS0513/1/1/ID 1567, Archives of the Royal College of Surgeons of England. For more information on Page, see Robert Burkett, Andrew England and Richard Rayner, 'Private Harold Page: A Norfolk Man', in *Stand To!*, the Journal of the Western Front Association (no. 106, 2016).

A triage system, known with brutal army logic as 'the preservation of effectives', was used to separate the wounded into three categories: men who after treatment would be able to return to the front lines; men like Page with severe but survivable wounds; and those whose wounds were so serious that they were unlikely to live. Those judged fit to return to combat soon were treated at the Base Hospital, but severely wounded men, including Page, who would require lengthy surgery and recuperation were sent back across the Channel for treatment.

On 6 July, five days after he had been wounded, Page arrived at the Cambridge Military Hospital in Aldershot, where he came under the care of Harold Gillies. Patients often arrived still wearing their battlefield uniforms and with filthy bandages covering their wounds. The heavily fertilized farmland, the mud, the stagnant water, the lack of sanitation and the plagues of rats and flies on the Western Front made infection a constant risk. Wounded men were less likely to die from their actual injuries than from infection and complications including tetanus, sepsis and 'gas gangrene', a rapidly progressing and life-threatening form of gangrene caused by Clostridium bacteria found in manure-enriched soil infecting an open wound. The infection caused toxins to form in tissues, cells and blood vessels, leading to necrosis (death) of the tissues, accompanied by the release of the foul gas that made the tissue crackle under an examiner's hand and gave the disease its name.

In an attempt to prevent infection, the first priority was to carry out a thorough cleaning and debridement of Page's wounds with an antiseptic solution, before applying fresh dressings. Gillies' clinical notes on Page recorded that his injury was a 'GSW (Gunshot Wound) right eye and cheek. A large lacerated wound involving practically the whole of the right face and right eye. Much necrosing tissue and blood clot about. Right eye has pus in anterior chamber. Right facial paralysis complete. Eye specialist recommends removal right eye.'

The work of stabilizing the wound and preparing to rebuild Page's face began at once, but sadly his right eye was so badly damaged that four days later, on 10 July, Gillies 'enucleated right optic' – removed Page's right eye.

After allowing time for his patient to recover his strength, Gillies carried out the first of a series of operations to restore Page's face to as much of its previous appearance and function as possible. He began to close the facial wound by advancing a flap from the cheek towards the nose, inserted a piece of celluloid to support the right side of the nose and closed the hollow left by the bullet wound on the right cheek with skin flaps that were sutured together. In the final stage of this first operation, pus was drained from the ethmoid sinus in the inner corner of the right eye socket.

Page was again allowed to recover for several months before Gillies performed another operation on him, in March 1917, to complete the full closure of the wound on his face by extending a flap upwards from the cheek to the bridge of the nose. Although the gaping wound had now been completely covered by grafts, Page was still badly disfigured and had much residual facial scarring and a badly deformed right eye socket. However, he was then discharged from hospital and allowed to recuperate at his home in Norfolk for over a year.

In August 1918 he was readmitted, and Gillies carried out a further operation on him. He harvested cartilage from Page's lower ribs but stored it under the skin, ready to be used later when reconstructing the upper jaw. Gillies did so because the free cartilage would not have survived being immediately transplanted into the damaged and scarred area of the face. Instead he used this method so that the cartilage could establish a new blood supply in a healthy area of the body and could then be transferred into the patient's face on the soft tissue and blood vessels now supplying it. At the same time, Gillies raised a cheek flap to reshape the corner of Page's right eye and enlarged the eye socket by easing over it the scar tissue that had left it misshapen and noticeably smaller than the left eye socket.

After a further three-month period of recuperation, in November 1918 the stored cartilage was removed and inserted under Page's right cheekbone and below the eye socket, providing a framework of solid tissue to build up the right side of his face. Two months later, Gillies further reshaped Page's right eye socket, constructed a lower eyelid, and sculpted the outer corner of the eye to give it a more normal appearance.

After constructing a new lining for Page's eye socket, Gillies inserted a prosthetic glass eye, and Page was discharged from hospital on 15 March 1919. Two years later, Gillies reassessed him. He was certainly contemplating further surgery to complete the restoration of Page's appearance, but in fact the ex-soldier never returned for further treatment. It was not uncommon for Gillies' patients themselves to call a halt to their treatment, even if their perfectionist maxillofacial surgeon was not yet satisfied, and Page may well have wanted to avoid the physical and psychological trauma of further operations, having evidently decided that his appearance was now good enough. The fact that he later got married suggests that he might well have been right.

We still use adaptations of the techniques Gillies pioneered in such treatments.

Just as in Harold Page's case, Gillies planned every procedure, extending through as many as half a dozen separate operations, with meticulous care. The method to be used was set out in the finest detail, and photographs and plaster casts were then made of the patient's face. Exact replicas of the areas of skin to be excised and grafted were cut from pieces of linen, and Gillies also calculated the exact dimensions of the tubed pedicles to be raised. Outlines were then drawn on to the patient's skin using a pen and 'Bonney's Blue' – a non-tattooing blue-green dye. Gillies was an artist as well as a brilliant technician, delicately and precisely handling his patients' tissues himself and demanding equal care from the rest of his team. Indeed he sometimes drove his assistants mad with his fanatical attention to detail and relentless striving for perfection, and was known to undo all the dozens of stitches he had already inserted if he felt that it was necessary to correct an error, even though it was so minuscule that only he was able to detect it.

He was swift and decisive when he needed to be but, as his motto 'never do today what you can honourably put off till tomorrow' suggested, he was a firm advocate of not rushing into action when it was not necessary. He was also a character with a quirky sense of humour that baffled many of his underlings, and a fondness for elaborate practical jokes. On one occasion he told his friends he was unable to join them on a golfing break, but that a South African colleague would be taking his place. He then turned up in plus fours and a tweed cap with a bushy false beard obscuring most of his face. His disguise fooled his friends completely and he was only rumbled several hours later, when he was given away by his mannerisms, particularly the way he smoked his cigarette after dinner, holding it between his second and third fingers. Gillies smoked like a chimney, even during the 'close' stages of an operation, and if any of his staff had the temerity to draw his attention to the column of ash dangling from the end of his cigarette that was about to fall on the patient, he would dismiss their concerns with a brusque 'Don't worry, it's perfectly sterile.'

He could be irascible, and a harsh critic of his subordinates when they failed to meet his exacting standards, but he always followed such criticism with kind and constructive advice on ways they could improve their skills. He was also very generous with his knowledge, sharing his techniques willingly and training countless surgeons from all over the British Empire in plastic surgery.

Gillies had inexhaustible energy and ingenuity, and an insatiable intellectual curiosity that was not always confined to the ways he could improve the techniques and equipment used in plastic surgery. In his spare moments he also devised an electric suction razor that he described as 'a cross between a dermatome [a knife for shaving off areas of the skin] and a vacuum cleaner'; he invented a revolving car seat that made it easier for people to get in and out of cars; and having observed that men always put on their trousers before their jackets when the design of coat hangers required them to take their jacket off the hanger to get at the trousers underneath, he designed an improved form of hanger with the trousers in front of the jacket.

Gillies' remarkable work on Harold Page and thousands of other disfigured patients won him international recognition as the world's pre-eminent surgeon in his field. He was mentioned in dispatches twice during the war, awarded an OBE in 1919, and a CBE the following year, and was knighted in the Birth-day Honours list of June 1930. The astonishing success he and his fellow surgeons enjoyed in rebuilding the bullet-, blast- and shrapnel-ravaged faces of the patients in their care is perhaps best reflected in one remarkable statistic: of the 11,752 major operations carried out at Sidcup between August 1917 and June 1921, only ten of the horrifically wounded men they treated proved to be so badly mutilated that even Gillies' remarkable skills could not restore their looks. These unfortunates were ultimately designated by the Ministry of Pensions as being 'incurably disfigured'. Even then, Gillies' team produced facial masks for them, covering their injuries and allowing them to go out in public without provoking revulsion and even horror in onlookers.

The publication of Gillies' ground-breaking book *Plastic Surgery of the Face* in 1920 cemented his reputation as the world's foremost practitioner of maxillofacial surgery. His fame also brought him many rich and famous private patients, including King Leopold of Belgium, who was treated for two separate injuries. More remarkably, Gillies also replaced a boy's missing ear, severed in an accident and damaged beyond use, by successfully transplanting an ear donated by the boy's maternal grandmother. The case was treated by the press as a near miracle, but Gillies' thorough research had already estab-lished the suitability of tissue from a close relative for use in transplants.

He also pioneered purely cosmetic surgery, including tech-niques for face-lifting. But he did nothing to promote them for several years, fearing – probably correctly – that if he did so he would be dismissed as a lightweight and a mere 'beauty surgeon' by his surgical peers. Only when his role as a supreme surgeon and surgical innovator was beyond dispute did he begin to carry out purely cosmetic procedures. When he still found himself challenged by critics claiming that such work was both 'unethical and unnecessary', Gillies responded, 'Is it not justified if it brings even a little extra happiness to a person who well needs it?' He offered the following sagacious and humorous advice to other cosmetic surgeons about what to do when meeting prospective patients for the first time: 'Avoid breaking the conversation with "And what would you like me to do to that huge nose, sir?" just as he is about to show you his Dupuytren's [a contraction of the hand, causing the fingers to bend towards the palm – also known as 'Thatcher's Claw' since the late Prime Minister suffered from it]!' Gillies later developed techniques in another controversial surgical area, by carrying out the first ever male-to-female and female-to-male gender reassignments.

In 1930 he was elected to the role of Consulting Plastic Surgeon at Barts – the hospital's first ever consultant in plastic surgery – and his justifiable pride in his own achievement was equalled by his pleasure at this recognition of the speciality he had developed. Gillies also took his nephew Archibald McIndoe under his wing. Another very gifted surgeon, McIndoe succeeded Gillies as Consultant Surgeon to the RAF in 1938, and when the Second World War broke out, while Gillies was supervising the setting up of mobile plastic surgery units in various theatres of the war, McIndoe became almost as famous as his uncle by restoring the ravaged faces of members of what was called 'The Guinea Pig Club', many of them airmen who had been disfigured by burns or wounds.

In 1957, thirty-seven years after publishing *Plastic Surgery of the Face*, Gillies drew on the meticulous records, case files, drawings and photographs he had accumulated and preserved in the course of his long career and used them as the basis of his masterwork, *The Principles and Art of Plastic Surgery*, which, over sixty years later, remains the definitive work. He died on 10 September 1960. A blue plaque on the wall of 71 Frognal in Hampstead, where he lived for many years, commemorates his remarkable life. While I was living in Hampstead and working at the Royal Marsden Hospital, I passed that sign every morning on my way to work and always drew fresh inspiration from it.

5

BEFORE BEGINNING TO read Medicine I had to complete my dental qualifications with a year as a houseman at Glasgow Dental Hospital, followed by a year as senior houseman at Newcastle General. The Geordies were lovely people to look after, 'like the Scots with the brains bashed out' as they used to say in Scotland, though Geordies probably thought it was the other way round. Working in A & E on a Saturday night, I certainly saw plenty of people who qualified for that description. It had a considerable impact on me because even though I'd grown up in a wee town with some ragged edges and had experience of rough areas of Glasgow, the sight of those Geordies in A & E with facial trauma – and 55 per cent of all serious facial trauma is the result of assault, while 80 per cent is alcohol-related – made me far more apprehensive about walking the streets of Newcastle late at night than I had ever been in Glasgow. Severe facial trauma was my first experience of the North East, before I had even seen the city properly. I knew there was no logic in it, but that didn't make the fear any less real to me.

I've always considered that poverty and unhappiness plus alcohol is a recipe for inter-personal violence – just another consequence of socio-economic deprivation. There was certainly plenty of evidence to support that hypothesis in both Glasgow and Newcastle in the early 1990s. I vividly remember the first time I was summoned to the A & E in Newcastle, at six in the morning, to examine a man who had been given a real pasting. He reeked of alcohol and had a very swollen face, lacerations, cuts, bleeding, bruises and abrasions, but there was no clear evidence of any bone injury on any of the scans. You wouldn't keep someone in hospital with just a cheekbone fracture anyway. Nonetheless, the guy was in a real state so I phoned the on-call registrar and said, 'I really think I should admit this guy because he's been given such a kicking.'

'Have you cleared his head injury?'

'I have, and I can't see any clear evidence of bone injury, but he's very swollen and sore.'

'Well, we're not a doss-house for drunks, so send him home.'

That seemed a bit harsh to say the least, especially as one of the problems with those kinds of cases is that, if they're still intoxicated, you can't really assess whether their mental state is caused by alcohol or head injury. So you should really keep them under observation until you're sure. But since I was only a houseman and he was a registrar, I did as I was told and sent the patient home.

The registrar may well have been right of course, and sometimes it is best to let nature take its course. One of the emergency medicine consultants at Newcastle used to complain that the patients in Intensive Care were often suffering from 'a lack of neglect', by which he meant that if you left them alone their problems would often solve themselves, while some interventions seem unhelpful – and there is a certain wisdom in that.

The unit at Newcastle was not the most cutting edge at the time, but there was enough contact with patients and with facial trauma and deformity surgery for me to be absolutely certain that maxillofacial surgery was what I wanted to be doing.

I had been offered a place at medical school in Glasgow and turned up at the anatomy lab on day one, a twenty-five-year-old surrounded by eighteen- and nineteen-year-olds straight from school. Revelling in the freedom of living away from home for the first time in their lives, as first- and second-year students tend to do, some would be saying 'It's Tuesday, let's get pissed', and I'd be countering with, 'Tell you what, let's not. Let's do the studying first and then we can revisit the Tuesday thing.'

The first operation I ever saw was back in 1987, during the Christmas break, while I was a second-year undergraduate student at dental school. It was in the Royal Alexandra Hospital in Paisley, where the father of my then girlfriend was a consultant hand surgeon and, knowing my interest in becoming a surgeon, he let me observe a procedure. The patient, a man called Archie, had punched his fist through a window while very drunk. The window hadn't disintegrated and dropped out of the way like you see them do in the movies, but instead had broken into jagged fragments, most of which were still attached to the frame. As he pulled his hand back through the hole he'd made, he'd caught his hand on a piece of this glass and it had sliced right through the extensor tendon on the back of his hand, paralysing his fingers.

As students we had been walked through the deserted operating theatre suite one morning as part of a tour of the hospital, but this was the first time I had ever been inside the theatre when an operation was in progress. It was a strange yet curiously familiar scene because, like everyone else, I had seen it so many times on the TV in hospital dramas. But this time it was real, and I drank it all in: the brilliance of the lighting, the smell of the anaesthetic, the beeping of the machines, and the patient, Archie, covered by surgical drapes, lying unconscious on the operating table with a big bandage, stained crimson by the blood he'd lost, covering his right hand. He was clearly something of a character because he had what looked like a homemade tattoo on his forearm, which read I LOVE BEV, though the grog blossoms and ruptured veins decorating his nose suggested that it was less likely to be in celebration of a woman named Beverley than of his fondness for a bevvy.

As the theatre nurse unwound the blood-encrusted bandage, she discovered that the last few inches were stuck firmly to the wound and she gave it a tug. As it came away with a tearing sound, Archie's back arched and his arm jerked upwards in a pain reflex. In alcohol-dependent or alcoholic persons – as was clearly the case with Archie – the brain becomes so used to the effect of depressant drugs that anaesthetics are less effective on them than they would be on less heavy drinkers. I had learned that from my lectures, but it was the first time I had seen it demonstrated in real life, though neither the anaesthetist nor the surgeon appeared to have registered the patient's discomfort – or if they had, they paid no attention to it. The surgeon simply peered at the wound and said, 'You'd better give that a wee scrub, nurse.'

The nurse picked up a smaller-scale, sterile version of a domestic scrubbing brush and went to work on the wound. Once more Archie responded to the pain with a repeat performance, arching his back and jerking his arm up. The nurse gave the surgeon a look that seemed to say 'Oh for God's sake', and he chortled in response.

I found it rather less amusing. The operating theatre suddenly became very much hotter and brighter; the sounds seemed to be coming from further and further away, and I felt my vision blur and fade. The last thing I heard as I started to topple was the scrub nurse yelling 'Don't touch that!' as I slumped towards a trolley laden with sterile instruments.

When I came round, a different nurse was checking me for signs of concussion and a burly porter with a very knowing grin on his face was holding my legs up to increase the venous return to my heart. Vasovagal or neurocardiogenic syncopy – fainting, as it's also called – happens when the body overreacts to emotional distress by reducing your heart rate. The blood vessels in your legs dilate, allowing blood to pool there, and your blood pressure falls to the point where it is inadequate for brain function, and you pass out.

I was mortally embarrassed. At the sight of a drop or two of blood and a couple of involuntary movements from a semi-anaesthetized patient I'd passed out right in front of a consultant surgeon. The fact that he was also my girlfriend's father only added to my humiliation. In my defence I can only say that it followed a night out in which rather more fluids than solids had been consumed, so I wasn't in the most sparkling of conditions even before the procedure began.

Once the nurses were satisfied that I wasn't going to keel over again the second they got me upright, I was taken out of the theatre and given a coffee with a couple of spoonfuls of sugar, and a piece of shortbread. I soon felt more human and made it back into the theatre for the end of the operation. I was still mortified, but captivated by what I'd seen of the procedure.

That was my first taste of the sharp end of surgery, but because of my fainting fit I hadn't actually seen that much, and the first time I actually saw human skin being cut was the following year, when I watched a senior surgeon operating on a patient who had suffered facial fractures, including a broken lower jaw. Such was the bone damage that the surgeon needed to make an external approach to the injury, by cutting into the neck beneath the jawline. As I waited for him to start, every one of my nerve-ends was tingling with anticipation and every sense was on maximum alert. It felt like that moment in *Jaws* when Roy Scheider suddenly realizes that there's a shark in the water and the cameraman jump-cuts right in on his face.

As I soon learned, first from watching other surgeons at work and later from doing it myself – and there really is no other way to replicate the feel of cutting through human skin than by actually doing it – you do not make an incision by cutting down and pressing on the skin with your blade. If you apply too much pressure or if your scalpel is less than super-razor sharp, the skin may pucker, making the incision less accurate, and unpredictably cutting the tissue below. The key is to generate tension in the epidermis which the blade then releases, by gently stretching the skin with the fingers of one hand and then applying the scalpel with the other. It's a delicate process, and when you do it correctly it feels more like painting a line on a canvas than slicing through it. Done well, there should only be minimal bleeding at this point.

As long as the blade is sharp, the knife just passes through the skin with barely any pressure, but the keratin layers of human skin blunt even the sharpest scalpel blade surprisingly quickly. It seems counter-intuitive because human skin is so soft and pliable to the touch and the blades that surgeons use are stainless steel and could not be sharper, yet you might make a single cut of no more than a few centimetres in length and then have to throw that scalpel away and reach for another because the

fineness of its edge has already been compromised. I've sometimes used as many as 140 scalpels in a single major operation.
Working in an era before disposable scalpels had been invented,
that was a luxury Harold Gillies was never granted.

The first incision to the neck exposes the bright, shining
layer of subcutaneous fat. Beneath it lies the orange-brown
platysma muscle, running from the upper chest to the chin,
and then comes the external jugular vein, from the angle of the
jaw down to the collarbone. The first time I witnessed at first
hand each layer being peeled back was the most mesmerizing
voyage of discovery. My senses were so finely tuned that I
noticed every detail, no matter how subtle or slight. Under the
glare of the overhead lights, the myriad colours glistened and
the blood showed bright crimson against the pure white of
the swab.

The first time I ever saw a flap raised was while I was on
placement from medical school. I knew the max fax (maxillofacial) team fairly well by then and heard they were in theatre
with a DCIA (Deep Circumflex Iliac Artery) case, using part of
the hip bone to repair a defect in a patient's jaw. So I got into
scrubs and went into the theatre. One surgeon was raising the
hip flap while another was preparing the 'top end', and what
was striking about the procedure to me was the sight of the
whole lateral abdomen being opened up. I hadn't seen that
before, and it was a huge incision. The layers of the abdominal
wall looked like bits of bread popping out of the top of a toaster
and flopping one way or the other, and it was fascinating to see
this massive hole being opened in the patient's stomach. It was
definitely a big step up from jaw fractures and teeth extraction,
and it was both exciting and absolutely terrifying to realize that

my colleagues and friends could already do that and that shortly I'd be expected to be able to do it too.

The atmosphere of the theatre was very new to me then. I wasn't used to the brilliant white light – so strong you can't even take a good photograph without moving or dimming the lights – and the bustle and activity of two surgical teams, two scrub teams and the anaesthetists. There was a constant dialogue between surgeons, anaesthetists and scrub nurses, punctuated by the metallic noise of implements being picked up and put down, all set against the beat of the background music. If you closed your eyes, you could almost imagine that you were in a car repair workshop, except that it smelled of tissue and blood, not petrol and engine oil.

I had some inspiring teachers and mentors at medical school, including Dr McDougal, a consultant obstetrician and gynae-cologist who taught me in my final year when I was doing obstetric work. He was not a great respecter of rules and regula-tions, and although smoking was not permitted in any NHS building, of course, he would take me into his office while he grabbed a sneaky cigarette break, keeping the window wide open to disperse the fumes. We would sit and chat while he smoked and he would keep me richly entertained with scurril-ous tales and anecdotes from his past. He didn't exactly tell his stories the way Dave Allen used to, but he certainly smoked his cigarette the way the old Irish comedian did, quietly pausing while he took a drag on his fag, and blowing the smoke into the air before delivering the punch line.

One of his tales, which could have come straight from the script of *Carry On Doctor*, was about the time when he and a colleague were training new doctors in the old Rotten Row hospital in Glasgow. They were living in the doctors' residence at the time and enjoying a very active social life. One weekend they held a particularly boisterous soirée, attended by other medical staff and a few nurses, one of whom spent the night with Dr McDougal. The morning after – though it was probably closer to the afternoon – he was leaving the building with the aforementioned nurse, doing the walk of shame, when the matron in charge of the doctors' residence threw open a first-floor window, stuck her head out and shouted down to him, 'Dr McDougal, did that young lady sleep here last night?'

At that, with a delivery of which even Kenneth Williams would have been proud, he smiled up at her and called out, 'Not a wink, Matron, not a wink.'

He was a real character and taught me lots of things (about medical matters, not entertaining nurses) that have stayed with me through my career; for instance, long before reflective practice became accepted as an important part of what we do, he took the time to sit in his office and chat with me about the day's events and the patients we'd seen. He had a very human and humane approach to patients and a lot of worldly-wise life experience, but at the time he was approaching the end of his long career. He'd had a stroke and had some numbness down one side of his body, but was able to carry on working despite that. Even though I was still an undergraduate, he always referred to me as 'Dr Jim' – as far as I could tell, without a hint of sarcasm – and I enjoyed working with him very much. He had a warmth in his approach with patients which, although very necessary, is not something all doctors possess, and he also had an interesting take on some disorders, such as somatization anxiety neurosis – the manifestation of psychological distress through physical symptoms. There is a spectrum of disorders where such distress affects the higher centres of the brain. It is perceived by patients as discomfort in another part of the body, whereas in fact that part of the body has no pathology affecting it; indeed it can even be absent, as it would be after a traumatic amputation. Dr McDougal sought a holistic understanding of people who came to his clinic, rather than simply looking for a diagnosis for which there was an automatic drug. I learned from him the importance of really listening to a patient and being seen to take on board what he or she is saying, because much of empathetic medicine is about how you *are* with people, rather than just reaching for a prescription pad.

Another clinician who made a big impact on me was Ross Lorimer, Professor of Medicine at Glasgow Royal Infirmary, for whom I worked as an 'intensive' – the term given to a student who is at the end of his training and has had concentrated medical exposure. And you certainly got that at Glasgow Royal Infirmary, which served the 'Wild East' of the city. He told me and his other students something that I still say to all my juniors today: one of the most important pieces of information we gain from our patients is their social history.

The first key thing to discover is who they live with at their home. Asking that question establishes the circumstances in which they are surviving, which is of particular importance, for example, if we are trying to plan 'day case' surgery, where the patient arrives at hospital in the morning for an operation and is then discharged the same day. We can carry out general anaesthetic procedures on them and send them home again the same day as long as two factors are fulfilled: there has to be a competent adult at home overnight to look after them, and there has to be a working telephone in the house, in case of a sudden emergency. Someone who normally lives on their own obviously has to make special arrangements. Equally, if a patient lives with an elderly parent for whom they are the main carer, it can be very problematic to admit that person for day case surgery, or indeed for a longer treatment, unless alternative care arrangements for the parent have been put in place. Asking that preliminary question also has the advantage of flushing out the patient's marital status, partner status, or other status, while avoiding a series of tricky questions that could seem too probing, intrusive and impertinent.

Professor Lorimer's message to his students, and it was one I took to heart, was that all these pieces of information about a patient's social history are absolutely essential in order to have a proper insight into the background and environmental causes that led to the illness. It also gives us an understanding of the life circumstances under which that person is coping and surviving, sometimes comfortably, sometimes not comfortably at all – as was often the case when treating patients from the East End of the city at Glasgow Royal Infirmary.

My studies, and my tutors, also taught me the vital importance of passing on skills and experiences from one generation of surgeons to the next, because hard-won knowledge should never be lost, in any discipline, but especially when people's lives are at stake.

6

BY THE TIME I had completed three years at medical school I was already married with an eighteen-month-old son, James, born in October 1994. I'd first met my future wife, Lorna, when we were both at dental school. I was in my third year and Lorna her fifth and final year. One night, just before Christmas, I heard on the grapevine that a medical insurance firm had put £200 behind the bar for the final-year students to enjoy a big night out. It was a decent sum of money in 1988 and I decided that the young fifth years might need a helpful third year like me to assist them in spending it. I'd recently fractured a meta-carpal and had my hand in plaster, which caught the attention of the tall, beautiful blonde with very straight hair who was standing next to me at the bar, waiting to be served. She looked at my hand and said, 'So, what happened to you?'

That was Lorna, and that was the start of something big. We spent the whole of that evening chatting and I scored points with her because she was from Dingwall, a small town in the Highlands, and I was one of the few people she'd met who actually knew where it was. Then we mainly talked about music and how when you hear something extraordinary it makes the hairs on the back of your neck stand on end. Listening to her speak had the same effect on me but, seeing that I'd only just met her, I didn't say so.

I had a great time, but I figured that being two years behind her I didn't really stand a chance, especially as we were going our separate ways for the Christmas holidays the next morning. But when I bumped into her in the corridor after returning to the dental school early in the new year, she gave me a dazzling smile and said, 'If you fancy going out some time, don't be scared to ask.' I did ask her. We began going out, fell in love, and got married in 1993.

As well as being my life partner, Lorna, a Specialist Consultant in Restorative Dentistry and Oral Rehabilitation, often works with me on cases where a patient requires a prosthesis to replace missing teeth after having part of their jaw removed. Once the transplanted bone has healed into its new site, Lorna uses a software CAD/CAM (Computer Aided Design and Computer Aided Manufacturing) package like Simplant to allow virtual placement of implants, then constructs a surgical stent – an acrylic guide – that clicks over the bone that has been surgically exposed in the mouth. She then uses 'guide chimneys' to drill down with precision into the underlying bone, so that the replacement teeth can be secured into the jawbone. The drill is centrally cooled with saline running up through the handpiece and into the centre of the burr, or drill-bit. That stops the bone from heating up – which is vital, because if the temperature reaches 46°, around 10° above normal body temperature, it causes the death of bone cells and prevents healing.

By 1996, as well as acquiring general medical skills, I was pursuing my interest – though Lorna would probably have said it was an obsession – in maxillofacial surgery. As a result, alongside my other studies, I was doing locum work in the evenings, at weekends and in any other spare time, developing my skills by working alongside the consultants at Canniesburn

Hospital in Glasgow and Monklands Hospital in North Lanark-shire. Lorna was also working three days a week, as well as doing the lion's share of child care.

In the spring of that year I applied for and won a T. C. White Travelling Fellowship from the Royal College of Physicians and Surgeons in Glasgow, enabling me to fly out to Miami in the summer to study gunshot trauma. One of the main reasons for this was that we'd just treated the victim of a shooting – an exceedingly rare event in the UK at the time. An eleven-year-old boy and his eight-year-old sister had been helping their father and uncle who were renovating a friend's ground-floor flat in a village just outside Glasgow when two masked men armed with shotguns approached the building. The two men let fly with both barrels through the window of the room. The boy, his father and uncle and the family friend were all peppered with shot, but the boy was the most serious casualty, sustaining wounds to his face, chest, arms and shoulder that were likely to leave him scarred for life and with permanent damage to his arm; his father had used his body to shield his daughter from the blasts and she'd escaped uninjured. The victims were rushed to hospital in Glasgow, where the boy underwent emergency surgery. A policeman was stationed outside the ward in case the gunmen came back to finish the job.

The car used by the two assailants was found burned out a couple of miles from the village. Neither of the boy's parents would make any comment to the press about the attack but it later emerged that his father was a prominent figure in the Glasgow underworld, and might well have been the intended target of the shooting as part of a long-running feud between two rival gangs. Soon afterwards, a man was murdered in the city in what was believed to be a revenge killing for the shotgun attack.

Gang violence had been a part of Glasgow life for as long as anyone could remember, from the Gorbals razor gangs in the 1920s who earned Glasgow the nickname 'Scar City', and the young thugs who ruled the concrete wastelands of Castlemilk and Easterhouse in the 1960s and 1970s using 'shivs' (knives or cut-throat razors) against their rivals and threatening anyone who strayed on to their turf, to the notorious 'ice cream wars' of the 1980s, in which battles were fought between gangs using ice cream vans as a front to cover the sale of drugs and stolen goods. Wars between rival gangs continue to this day.

But this shotgun case, and another in which we treated a victim who still had the bullet lodged in his head, led to a general discussion about improving the way we dealt with gunshot trauma. I was determined to improve my knowledge of the most effective ways to treat such wounds. In the First World War, Harold Gillies had made Britain a world leader in dealing with gunshot trauma, but surgical and medical techniques had moved on dramatically since his time. Britain was no longer at the forefront, because other countries, notably the United States, not only had troops involved in regular combat, but a weapon-owning culture that made gunshot injuries an everyday occurrence in its major cities. As a result, US surgeons had become the acknowledged experts in dealing with gunshot trauma.

In the mid-1990s the use of firearms was growing in the UK – the principal reason why I felt the need to improve my skills in dealing with the consequences – but there just weren't enough victims of gun crime to treat. Even now, bullet wounds are a rarity, whereas in the USA, guns and the injuries and deaths they cause were and are of pandemic proportions. In 2013, for example, the US Center for Disease Control and Prevention reported a total of 117,894 shootings: 84,258 non-fatal injuries and 33,636 deaths due to 'injury by firearms' (including homicides, suicides and deaths due to accidental discharge of a firearm). That is about one death every fifteen minutes, day and night throughout the year, and the annual rate of deaths was over forty-five times that of the UK. Even more relevant to my field of work was the fact that one in five of all those gunshot injuries were wounds to the face.

I chose to work in Miami because, even by American standards, its rate of violent crime was very high – almost three times the US national average – so facial trauma from gunshot wounds was, and still is, a daily occurrence. I'd been in regular communication with Tim O'Keeffe, the senior chief resident in the maxillofacial surgical training programme at Miami's Coral Gables Hospital, and I was staying with him but working with Dr Robert E. Marx, a consultant who was well known for his work on using hyperbaric oxygen to prevent or reduce osteoradionecrosis (chronic damage to the bone from radiotherapy).

Tim drove me to his house and introduced me to his wife, Margy, and baby son. Like Lorna, Margy was a dentist whose speciality, endodontics (the branch of dentistry concerned with diseases of the dental pulp), was one of the three areas covered by Lorna's speciality, restorative dentistry. Her other claim to fame was that she had once treated the American baseball legend Joe DiMaggio, and she had the pictures to prove it. They lived in a gated community with access through the guarded main gate via swipe card. I didn't find the razor wire along the top of the perimeter walls a particularly reassuring sight, but at least the community was far enough out of Miami – or so Tim assured me – that there was no danger of my sleep being disturbed by gunfire.

As I discovered on my first solo excursion beyond the gate, if you didn't have a swipe card and couldn't remember the four-digit code – and I'd already managed to forget both of them – the guard on the gate would not allow you in, no matter how much you pleaded. 'Sure I recognize you, doctor,' he said when I pointed out that I'd already been in and out a couple of times with Tim, 'but I still can't let you in without the code.' Since he was wearing a side-arm – still an alarming sight to a Brit back then, though sadly we're much more used to them now – I didn't argue any more and retreated to a nearby Starbucks to wait for Tim to come and swipe me in.

After a good night's sleep, I went into the hospital with Tim early the next morning. We had a choice of two highways to get us to work. On one you paid a toll and there was never a sign of any police on it, but they were always all over the one that was toll-free. An incident while I was there – a real *Bonfire of the Vanities* scenario – demonstrated to me part of the reason for that. A German couple took the wrong exit, got lost and ended up in a cul-de-sac in a very rough, gang-ruled area. As they tried to reverse away, some of the gang members fired at them, and although the couple were unharmed, one bullet smashed through the windscreen, passed between the two of them and hit and killed their baby in the back seat. That terrible tragedy was a sobering warning to me that local knowledge was not just a luxury but an absolute necessity, and I quickly made sure that I memorized the route to the hospital.

The hospital at Coral Gables was a handsome, white, two-storey building set in beautiful gardens. You parked your own car, unlike at the maxillofacial unit at the University of Texas Medical School in Houston, where I've also had a brief residency, which had valet parking for surgeons (like the man said, 'Only in America!'). Coral Gables was very swish and very American, just like the hospitals I'd seen in countless dramas, with push-bar handles on the doors and a slightly different tang of antiseptic than I was used to in the UK. The hallway was lined with fresh flowers and the receptionists were very smiley and friendly, so all the 'front-facing peripherals' were present and correct, and the facilities were great.

The operating theatre was similar to UK ones, quite compact and equipped to a very high specification, though the wire-reinforced security glass in the windows was not a feature I'd ever seen at home. In my paranoia about the extent of gun violence in the area, albeit partly justified by those horrendous gun-crime statistics, I did catch myself wondering if even the operating theatre might not sometimes be under siege from armed gunmen. In the midst of so much that was different from a UK hospital, the scrubs we wore were reassuringly familiar. They were the same colour as at several hospitals I'd worked at in the UK, reinforcing my sneaking suspicion that purple is popular with hospital administrators mainly because purple scrubs don't get stolen as often as green or blue ones.

I had come to Miami to study gunshot trauma, and on my very first morning I had an opportunity to do so. All shooting incidents are tragic, but this case was particularly awful. It involved a ten-year-old boy – a nice middle-class kid from a nice middle-class home. While his dad was at work and his mom was doing something in the kitchen, the boy, bored, had been rooting around in a closet when he found his father's .357 Magnum. Made famous by Clint Eastwood's 'Dirty Harry' character, the Magnum is one of the most powerful handguns you can buy, designed to fire a round capable of penetrating car bodywork and bullet-proof vests, so its impact on fragile human flesh is absolutely devastating.

According to the boy, the gun had fallen out of the closet, hit the floor and gone off, blowing off his jaw and the front of his face. The resulting trauma was very similar to what sadly often happens when people attempt to commit suicide using a shotgun. The would-be suicide puts the shotgun under his chin, but as he reaches down for the trigger he unknowingly alters the angle of both his head and the gun-barrel, with the result that when he does pull the trigger, rather than kill himself he blows his jaw and the front of his face off instead. I have had to try and remedy the results of such tragic cases several times in the course of my surgical career.

Although the boy continued to claim that the gun had just fallen out of the closet, I suspected that he had been playing around with it and was holding it under his chin when it had gone off. The scans showed the full extent of the horrific defect caused by a round fired at point-blank range from a powerful Magnum, and the real surprise was that the wound was survivable at all. The results were bad enough: the boy had permanently lost sight in one eye and reconstructing his face was going to be a very long and painful process, involving a minimum of half a dozen separate operations.

Predictably enough, the story was just a five-minute wonder meriting no more than a couple of brief paragraphs in the local paper; equally predictably, a National Rifle Association spokesman was soon emerging from the woodwork to shoot down calls for the laws on gun ownership to be tightened ... just another day in America. The boy's treatment was still ongoing when I left Miami, but he was still facing yet more operations and yet more pain to restore as much normal appearance and function to his face as possible. However successful the surgery ultimately proved to be, he would be blind in one eye for the rest of his life and might well carry the psychological trauma of the incident, the surgery and people's reactions to his altered face with him to the grave.

Had that been an isolated, freak accident it would have been bad enough but my colleagues at Miami could point me to a string of similar incidents involving children, many of which had ended in even more tragic fashion. A few months earlier a four-year-old boy had accidentally killed himself with his adult cousin's Magnum. It had been put in a high cupboard but the doors had been left open, leaving the butt of the gun visible. The little boy, who according to his mother watched lots of 'cops and robbers' programmes on TV, had been intrigued enough to find a way to get to it. While his mother and his cousin were in another room, the little boy stacked a plastic baby chair on top of a baby seat and a box for a plastic Christmas tree, climbed up and reached the weapon. 'I guess he just wanted to see how the gun worked,' his mother said. 'He wanted to be a little gangster.' The gun went off, mortally wounding the little boy, who bled to death in his mother's arms.

Within a couple of months of that appalling incident an even younger boy, just thirty months old, shot himself with his father's .380 semi-automatic pistol and also died. Police and gun manufacturers issued a series of safety tips for gun owners with children, including the advice to fit a trigger lock to their weapon, keep it unloaded and store it and the ammunition in separate places, and if the gun was loaded, to keep it in a locked case or metal box. In the hope of preventing yet more accidental shootings when children discovered guns in their own homes, or those of their friends and families, the city of South Miami went even further than that, passing an ordinance requiring locks on all firearms stored within the city limits. However, since gun owners routinely cited protecting themselves, their families and their property against intruders as the principal reason for possessing a weapon, the idea that they would then leave themselves vulnerable by keeping it locked away, or with guns and bullets in separate places, seemed optimistic to say the least. The evidence of the ongoing carnage among Miami's children suggested that most gun owners continued to keep their weapons loaded and easily accessible, whether or not they were breaking the law by doing so.

So far, all my experience of gunfire and the trauma it caused had been achieved by viewing it from the wrong end of the barrel, so to speak. Although there was no medical or surgical need, nor probably any genuine justification for it, I was curious to know what it would be like to pull the trigger and see the impact of bullets for myself – though only on a target, not human flesh. So when the local police chief heard about my interest in studying the effects of gunshot trauma and invited me to see some of the handguns that had been used in crimes and fired at the police, and try one out on their firing range, I jumped at the chance. He also showed me a study conducted by the Firearms Department of the City of Miami Police Training

Unit to find the most appropriate ammunition to use in their .40-calibre Glock pistols, the weapon of choice for 65 per cent of all US law enforcement agencies, according to the company's promotional literature. Forty-calibre is the equivalent of about 0.4 inches in diameter, which makes the bullets the Glock fires pretty chunky.

The criteria the study took into consideration included:

1. Penetration. According to the FBI, a projectile must be able to penetrate soft body tissue to a depth of twelve inches in order to be effective.
2. Permanent cavity. The projectile should expand a cavity large enough to promote tissue destruction to create rapid bleeding in order to incapacitate the subject as rapidly as possible, therefore stopping the threat.
3. Fragmentation. In order to achieve maximum penetration and permanent cavity, the projectile should keep its integrity and not fragment.

That report, assessing gunshot trauma in such cool, calculated terms, made chilling reading. For example, at most angles of entry, the twelve-inch penetration required would take a projectile right through the human body and out the other side, blowing a substantial exit hole in the process, and also potentially wounding anyone behind them.

Having thoroughly put the wind up me, the police chief then took me down to the firing range under the building and let me fire one of their .40-calibre Glock pistols. He told me that most exchanges of gunfire in law enforcement happened at close range, inside buildings, and in the space of two or three seconds.

So the standard police practice drill, rather than standing and aiming at a target twenty-five metres away, is to wait until someone shouts 'Go!' and then fire two rounds into a close-range target as fast as possible – the 'double-tap' made famous by our own SAS. However, slightly to my disappointment, I was being given the easier option of a standard firing range target.

I'd never fired anything more threatening than an air rifle before and, having dressed to impress in a suit and a white shirt with a breast pocket, I felt more than a little conspicuous among my growing audience of hard-bitten law enforcement professionals, all wearing police uniform or sweatshirts and suitably sceptical and/or amused expressions. After a lengthy safety briefing, I put on a pair of ear-defenders and took my stance at the counter of one of the firing stalls, facing a paper target of a 'bad guy'. The police chief gave the laconic command 'Go get 'em, son', and I began firing.

Each time I fired, a round disappeared in the general direction of the target, while the spent casing was automatically ejected from the breech. But such was the heat generated by the act of firing that when one of the casings bounced off the partition on my right, ricocheted up on to the roof and then dropped with uncanny accuracy straight into my shirt pocket, the heat was so intense that it scorched the fabric and burned my nipple. That caused me to dance around in agony, still waving the loaded weapon in my hand, much to the consternation of the police who all stopped laughing and dived for cover, yelling, 'Don't point that f***ing thing at me!'

At the end of the firing range session the team trained me in the side-on stance, swift-arm-raise technique – like pointing a finger at the target individual and shooting at very close range.

That was a different and in many respects more alarming skill to develop, even though my 'human' target was only reinforced paper. I could feel the power of the recoil forcing back my arm and shoulder as the round exited the barrel, and in my mind's eye, rather than a paper target I could see the mangled faces of gunshot trauma patients. The smell of burned ammunition propellant remains a very emotive one for me because it is always associated in my mind with the coppery tang of fresh blood and the sight of blast-damaged human bone and soft tissue.

I learned a huge amount about treating gunshot trauma in the time I was in Miami. One of the first things I discovered there was that the muzzle velocity of handguns had dramatically increased in recent years, hugely complicating the work of repairing wounds caused by gunfire. Many older types of pistol had a muzzle velocity below the speed of sound in air – 300 metres per second – and the wounds they created were the product of 'low-energy transfer', caused by the bullet itself. However, modern pistols can create far more serious injuries because, depending on the weight and type of bullet, the muzzle velocity of a modern 9mm pistol ranges from 300 to as much as 540 metres per second. The 9mm Glock pistol, for example, has a muzzle velocity of 375 metres a second.

As well as the tissue damage caused by the primary missile (the high-velocity bullet itself) there is also a 'cavitation effect' because the bullet sucks in gas and superheats it with explosive effect inside the wound, forming an ellipse-shaped permanent cavity. Even worse, projectiles from such weapons produce wounds as a result of 'high-energy transfer' that are far more devastating than those from low-energy transfer. In the early stages of the First World War, massive tissue damage was caused by rounds fired from new types of rifle that even then had a velocity of over 300 metres a second. Although those bullets weren't producing quite the cavitation effect of a modern round, they were pretty close to it, and those effects – on a scale never seen before in battlefield casualties – led both sides to accuse each other of using explosive bullets or 'dum-dum' rounds.

At a velocity of over 300 metres a second, a projectile striking the mandible will shatter and fragment it and, just like shrapnel, those fragments will then become secondary projectiles, ripping through the soft tissues and causing massive additional damage to the face. While I was in Miami, we were treating a minimum of one victim of the effects of such shootings a day. Among the many I saw there was a young woman who had been withdrawing some cash from a drive-through ATM when an attacker with a gun tried to steal her money and her car. She floored the accelerator and sped off but as she did so the attacker fired at her. The bullet, coming from behind and on her right side, punched through the rear window, struck her in the neck, passed through the back of her cheek and smashed out through her jaw, creating the shrapnel effect that blew off the lower third of her face.

The 'first look' surgery on her was purely concerned with cleaning the wounds and removing the particles of shattered bone – and there were an awful lot of those. After the initial debridement of the wound, carefully preserving vital structures such as nerve and blood vessels where possible, we stabilized it by packing it with gauze soaked in an iodine solution. We then had to undertake a 'second look' procedure to debride necrotic tissue (soft tissue that had died because too little blood was flowing to it) before the definitive reconstruction could begin. It had already taken many days of treatment just to reach that stage. To redress that devastating and life-changing injury then required major surgery and several months of further treatment. It was ultimately successful, and I later shared with my American colleagues the joy of seeing that young woman, once so terribly disfigured, leave hospital with not just her face but her positive outlook on life fully restored.

After I got back, I wrote a major report for the Royal College of Physicians and Surgeons of Glasgow on what I had learned. Apart from the strengthened conviction that gunshot trauma is difficult to manage, one of the most important things I brought back was the need for delay when treating it. With gunshot wounds it really is important to wait and not rush into anything because what you see is often not what you get. The temptation is always to clean a wound and close it up, and when you're starting to work on a patient's face that has been torn apart by gunfire there's a temptation to start clamping blood vessels right, left and centre to stop the bleeding; but there are so many important structures in the face, such as facial nerves, sensory nerves and the nerves and muscles that control the movement of the eyeballs, that in cutting off the blood supply to them there is a risk of doing more harm than good.

So, rather than blindly clamping everything in an effort to stop the bleeding, as you might do with a limb, thorax or abdominal wound, it's much better to apply pressure and then get the patient to the operating theatre, where the wounds can be better evaluated and treated. The priority is to clean up and take away any dead material – tissue, muscle and bone fragments – but give a chance to anything that might still be viable.

We tend to pack the wounds with gauze soaked in iodine solution, leave it for forty-eight hours and then take another look when things have settled down a little, because tissue that initially looks OK often won't be with time due to the heat generated in the wound and the effect of the secondary missiles, the bone and tissue fragments. As a result of that, in complete contrast with cancer treatment where the tissue around the tumour is as viable as it's ever going to be, some of the soft tissue around the bullet wound that initially appeared healthy will necrose and cease to be viable, so you have to learn to pack the wound, wait, and then go back in.

People who get shot tend to be much younger and fitter than cancer patients, since cancer is a disease of ageing – for example, head and neck cancer peaks in the seventh and eighth decades of life – and the age of the patient has a major impact on their recovery. In a mouth or throat cancer patient it's also unusual for the disease to make much of a difference to how the face looks, unless it's very advanced and the patient may end up needing a patch of fascia and skin from their arm or leg on their face. But as I said, that's quite unusual, whereas, as the photographs of Harold Gillies' First World War patients demonstrate, a projectile just rips everything away. So there's a very different challenge in trying to put that back together, and the appearance is going to be very different. If you've got the facial skin intact, even if you've had to split it down the middle to excise a tumour, the scars can be hidden, whereas projectile wounds are almost always going to require a composite reconstruction involving bone and skin and muscle, or at the least two out of those three.

The need for speed in treatment is also different. With

cancer, even a delay of a few days in treating someone may be critical, whereas with gunshot wounds, once the airway has been made safe and the initial blood loss has been controlled, there is less reason to rush back to the operating theatre, and in fact there are good reasons not to. The reconstruction will take a lot of planning since there are so many important structures that need to be protected to maintain the proper functioning of the swallowing apparatus, salivary glands, the face muscles and everything else, and there is time to plan it.

If they survive the shooting itself, the prognosis for patients with gunshot wounds in the longer term is obviously a lot better than for cancer patients, but they may also have to come to terms with the reality of disfigurement, and since most gunshot victims are young, like that tragic ten-year-old boy in Miami playing with his father's Magnum .357, they will have to live with the consequences for many, many years.

Although, as a visitor from the UK, everybody was very polite to me in Miami, there was the language barrier for me to overcome. As George Bernard Shaw remarked, we are 'two countries divided by a common language', with the added complication that I have a strong Scottish accent. It did cause some communication issues, although mainly with people who were not expecting it and were a bit taken aback at first. I do tend to think quickly and speak quickly, and even in my native Scotland there are occasions, particularly if I'm tired, when I drop the volume of my voice and speak so fast that even fellow Scots are forced to ask, 'What the hell is he talking about?' However, as I always like to remind them, 'It's not that I'm speaking too quickly, it's just that you're thinking too slowly!'

As well as slight issues with my accent and the minor differences between our two countries' healthcare systems, there was one very significant discrepancy that took a lot of getting used to: unlike the NHS, the American system is not free at the point of need. As I went about my work, I was always struggling to suppress the unsettling question, 'What about all the people who can't afford this?' The system wasn't as bad as 'You feel for his pulse and I'll feel for his wallet', but I was aware that people who were fully insured had excellent healthcare available whenever it was needed, but there were an awful lot of uninsured or inadequately insured people around town who didn't.

I was given a vivid demonstration of this with a cancer patient, Irene, who was about to undergo surgery to replace the whole of her lower jaw. Instead of a free tissue transfer which we would tend to use now, the procedure the American consultant had chosen involved harvesting bone from the back of her hip – the posterior iliac crest. That was crushed in a bone mill, turning it into a sort of heavy paste, which was then mixed with platelet-rich plasma. Platelets are tiny cell fragments that form the initial plug when a blood vessel is damaged. Very significantly for the reconstructive surgeon, they also contain proteins that promote cell growth and healing. This is called Platelet Derived Growth Factor (PDGF).

To obtain the platelet-rich plasma, a unit of blood is taken from the patient and spun in a centrifuge to separate the red cells, which are then transfused back into the patient. The remaining blood, minus the red cells but containing the platelets, is then spun down again in the centrifuge, further concentrating the platelets. Clotting factors still present in the remaining fluid cause it to set when calcium chloride solution is added to it, setting off a 'coagulation cascade' to form a clot. The milled bone combined with the paste containing a very high concentration of platelets and PDGF forms a solid healed bone reconstruction. When implanting it, you have to drill into it slowly to keep it cool as you connect it to the existing jawbone to avoid those bone cells heating beyond 46°, at which point they necrose, but the concentrated PDGF gives a whole lot of growth factor to that bone, making for a really solid graft.

But the technique is only really useful for benign cases because, for obvious reasons, we don't like concentrating growth factor near cancer cells, so if there are any near the area we're treating, that is a problem. If it's a benign case, or damage of any other sort, then there is time to develop a soft tissue envelope at a much later stage when the soft tissues are all healed and then place the bone graft inside it, but that is not appropriate for cancer reconstruction, which has to be done immediately to prevent further spread of the disease, with life-threatening consequences.

When cancer has eaten into the facial bones, the only way to cure the disease currently is to remove the bone that has been violated by cancer cells. Radiotherapy, which normally wipes out the DNA in cells like a deadly laser beam in a black-and-white sci-fi movie, cannot penetrate far enough into the dense, calcified bone tissue to guarantee destruction of the cancer cells. Even when we remove the contaminated facial bone and the pathology doctor examines it under the microscope and confirms that the cancer has been completely removed, we know that this is not enough treatment to stop it returning. Radiotherapy is then mandatory because cancer cells that do have the ability to penetrate solid human bone tend to remain in microscopic, undetectable numbers in the surrounding soft tissues, even when the surgeon removes a tumour with a clear margin around it. The cancer cells then re-form into face-invading deposits which are often untreatable.

Another corollary of this need for radiation treatment is damage to the new bone transplanted into the face to reconstruct human facial shape, form and function. Although the radiation doesn't penetrate far enough into bone to destroy all the cancer cells it can contain, it does damage and weaken the bone. As a result, the new facial hard tissue (bone) that we've transplanted is far less able to withstand holes being drilled in it, even if we do so with meticulous care, and may not heal around an implant that has been placed in order to replace vital missing teeth, allowing the patient to smile and chew again. Sometimes, disastrously, this new facial tissue may necrose, causing intense pain and infection, and has to be removed to save the patient's life, leaving behind a gaping hole in the face. So we have to do facial reconstructions at the first cancer-removing surgery, before radiotherapy takes place. This must include placing titanium implants to allow a denture to be constructed and function to be recovered, at that first major operation. If a patient has had radiotherapy to their face first, it's very difficult to operate on it afterwards. Having said that, it's increasingly what we are required to do, because people have chemotherapy and radiotherapy to try to cure the cancer, and if that doesn't work, they then come to us to try to salvage their situation.

Accumulated therapy – surgery, followed by chemotherapy and radiotherapy – is a hard ask and patients quite often say, 'If I'd known what it was going to be like, I wouldn't have had it.' However, when one of my patients recently said that to me, I had to reply, 'I hear what you're saying, but do you know what? If you hadn't had the therapy, we wouldn't be having this conversation, because you wouldn't be here at all.'

Patients who are enduring the hair loss, the nausea, the exhaustion, the pain and all the other unpleasant, debilitating side-effects of their therapy also have one consolation that they should cling to: people who get the worst side-effects in the broadest sense are the ones who tend to have the best outcomes from the therapy. Individual humans have differing levels of radio sensitivity but the radiation dosages given are averaged, based on large clinical trials and their effects. There is a normal distribution across the range of people, so some suffer more side-effects than others, but if you have one group of people on a trial who report very severe side-effects and another who report almost no side-effects at all, the latter group is the one you would worry about in terms of treating their cancer. The reason is that cancer cells are always derived from normal tissue that has gone wrong, so there is a reasonably close symmetry between the sensitivity of your normal cells to radioactivity and that of your cancer cells. If your normal cells are not much affected by the radioactivity, and therefore do not produce much in the way of side-effects, that means that cancer cells will not be much affected by it either. So the consolation for those who suffer the worst side-effects is that they do so because their bodies are reacting strongly to the radiation, which means that its beneficial effects will also be greater for them than those who report having no or very few side-effects.

In the case of Irene in Miami who was about to have her lower jaw replaced, there was an additional problem that had nothing to do with medical complications. I was told that because of the terms of her insurance cover, she was not to be considered a hospital patient the night before the operation, but merely to be regarded as what was termed a 'hotel patient'. She was occupying a hospital bed and would be a hospital patient when the operation began the next morning, but I was firmly instructed that the night before the operation she was to be considered only as a guest occupying what was effectively a hotel room for the night.

As a result of that, when I went to see Irene that evening I was not permitted to prescribe her anything for the pain she was suffering. She had already taken all the medication she had with her but was still in a lot of discomfort, and had I been back in the UK I would simply have prescribed her the appropriate analgesia for pain relief, but in an American hospital I could not do that. Had I done so, both I and the hospital could have been open to litigation, and one thing I was already learning about the US was that, although if you weren't wealthy or insured you couldn't always be sure of obtaining medical treatment, no matter how poor you might be you could always be sure of finding a lawyer to sue someone for you.

As the realization that I could offer no palliatives for Irene's pain began to dawn on me, it was reinforced by my co-resident Steve Schimmele, a 'Hoosier' from Indiana with a broad Midwestern drawl who was normally quite a laugh. 'No way,' he said, as he saw me hesitating. 'You can't do it [prescribe medication].' As he spoke, I was very aware of the stillness and silence in the room, and the metallic tang of antiseptic in my mouth and nose seemed sharper than usual. Irene looked up at me and I could only gaze helplessly back at her before muttering some platitudes and then leaving her to endure a night of pain.

That whole experience was completely alien to me. The key to excellent medical care is knowing when you can make a change to benefit a patient, so it was an oddly helpless, empty feeling to know that I could have removed Irene's pain but was prevented from doing so by a healthcare system that ought to have had the same priorities. I felt that all my years of training and the power that conferred on me had been negated, not for medical reasons but to satisfy the requirements of the small print of an insurance policy. That incident remains fresh in my memory today, and whenever I hear people talk about moving to an American-style health system in this country – and it's something that right-wing politicians are increasingly open about advocating – the thought of that woman enduring a pain-racked night comes back to me.

7

WHEN I RETURNED from Miami I completed my basic medical training, emerging in 1997 with another honours degree, and as far as I know I'm still the only graduate from Glasgow University with honours in both Dentistry and Medicine – a tremendous springboard for my career. My fixed ambition was still to be a maxillofacial surgeon, so it was just a matter of going through all the required steps, but with a double qualification in both Dentistry and Medicine and then all the advanced medical and surgical training, it was a far from speedy process.

As part of our training, all medical students have to work as a junior houseman, continuing their education as the most lowly member of hospital medical or surgical teams. I'd already been a houseman at the end of my dental degree, but I now had to repeat the process as a junior medic. So I began as a houseman at Western Infirmary. By then I was twenty-eight going on twenty-nine, whereas the average houseman was usually twenty-two or twenty-three. So my seniors realized I had been around the block a bit more than my peers and gave me a little more responsibility as a result.

Houseman jobs are divided between general medicine and general surgery, and obviously, given my ultimate ambition, I preferred the latter path, although both were required of me. At the start, my work was mainly administrative, served with a side-dish of sleep deprivation. The job was ward-based and fairly grim, but you had to do it because only upon successful completion of that year did you become fully registered as a doctor with the General Medical Council.

I was working long shifts: all day, all night and all day again, and then back the following morning to do it all over again. It was unremittingly hard work, because if needed, we were also on call outside those already long hours. Although I sometimes work very long hours now, particularly when a procedure proves particularly challenging because the patient's general health is not good, his blood vessels are in poor condition, or his tissues and bone have been damaged by radiotherapy, such long days and nights are comparative rarities, whereas back then they were an everyday occurrence and the challenges were relentless as a succession of ill or injured patients passed through my hands.

I turned up in scrubs on day one to find 104 occupied beds. I hadn't met any of the patients and though there were nursing staff there, I didn't get to meet any of my fellow medics either at that stage: there was no hand-over because the day people had already gone home. So, having said hello to the nurses, there I was, wearing scrubs and trainers and in possession of two bleepers, trying to be a bit of a presence on the ward, but actually just standing there, waiting for stuff to happen – and with 104 patients to deal with, I knew I wouldn't have to wait long before something did. I spent my days and nights going around the ward, sometimes inserting intravenous cannulas into patients but mostly filling out paperwork and discharge prescriptions, and standing around while the more senior trainees did all the interesting stuff.

There were five floors of medical wards and it was a war zone in some respects, though there were some lighter moments too.

I had a spell helping to deliver babies in the maternity unit and it was thrilling to be involved in bringing new lives into the world. For obvious reasons most of the parents were even more excited, but one seasoned mother was surprisingly blasé. When I told her that she had a fine, healthy baby boy and asked her if she wanted to hold him, she thought about it for a couple of seconds, then said, 'No, you're all right, son. When can I get a fag?'

My surgical training started at a unit that treated many cases of breast cancer and had an acute receiving ward, which generally dealt with any patients complaining of abdominal pain. My job was really dull and purely clerical, filling out paperwork and barely getting to the operating theatre at all. I made it there just twice, and only then because I was so enthusiastic to see what was going on that I grabbed a chance to sneak down there. My arrival was greeted with a mixture of remarks: either 'Gosh, here's a keen one, what do you want to do?' or, less welcoming, 'What are you doing down here, and who's doing your job on the ward?'

One day I was allowed to assist in the removal of a kidney and learned a very valuable lesson. During the procedure, a clamp came off one of the patient's arteries, leading to an alarming gush of crimson, arterial blood. Even the consultant looked quite perturbed about that for a moment but he simply stopped the bleeding by pressing on the artery with his finger and then asked the scrub nurse for a stronger clamp. His cool, quick reaction showed me how important it is to be the calmest person in the room in those kinds of situations. If blood is whooshing everywhere, it is easy to panic or take a hasty action that might make the situation worse, whereas you can nearly always stick a hand or a finger on a bleeding blood vessel, slow or stop the flow and then think, 'OK, let's give some thought to what we're going to do now.'

If usually less dramatic than that, almost every case taught me something of value. Medical and surgical training is designed to help us make patients better, of course, but our training also has to prepare us for the inevitable occasions when, no matter how dedicated and skilled we are, nothing can prevent the death of the patient we are caring for.

Breaking bad news about a death, or cancer, or any other serious condition is a difficult and very delicate process. I was still a houseman when I discovered just how difficult it could be. A woman called Martha, who was in her early thirties, was brought in with bowel obstruction, distended stomach, absolute constipation, nausea, vomiting and abdominal pain. From the X-ray imaging and further investigation it became evident that she had ovarian cancer, extending into her abdomen. That gave us all a sinking feeling, but despite that the oncology team decided to attempt to treat her. However, before that could happen, the surgical team had to open part of her small bowel and attach to the abdominal wall an ileostomy bag, to stop waste passing from the ileum (small intestine) into the colon. As soon as she had recovered from that operation, the oncology team could begin her treatment.

The on-call room for the senior house officer, who oversees in-patient and emergency care and supervises the junior house officer, who is usually just out of medical school, was about 400 yards away, so in the intervals between emergencies when we could try to get a little rest most of us preferred to slip into a patient bed in an empty four-bedded side-ward on the floor above the surgical ward. In those days we had pagers, not mobile phones, and if we were bleeped we had to get up and go and see what the emergency was.

That night I was lying there, wearing my scrubs as pyjamas, with my trainers on the floor at the side of the bed, when my pager went off. I snoozed through the first alert, murmuring, 'I'm coming . . . I'm coming . . .' Then it went off again. Still not fully awake, I had swung my feet on to the floor and was working them into my trainers when the junior house officer appeared in the doorway. 'Jim! Jim!' she said. 'Come now. It's Martha.'

I looked blearily at my watch: four in the morning. I had already learned that cardiac arrests happen more frequently at that time than at any other because that's when the circadian rhythms are at their lowest level and the body is at its lowest ebb in its natural twenty-four-hour cycle. It's also when the doctors and nurses are at their lowest ebb. I ran downstairs and found that, sure enough, Martha had had a cardiac arrest.

Now a real cardiac arrest is quite unlike the depictions shown on TV, even in fairly modern dramas, in that, having had an in-hospital cardiac arrest, the chances of you leaving hospital as an intact and fully functioning human being are only around one in twelve. That may seem like a shockingly low recovery rate given instant access to trained staff and all the necessary equipment, but the reason for it is a simple one. Anyone who is already in hospital when they have a cardiac arrest is there because they are very sick anyway and usually their heart has stopped because of other problems that need to be fixed, otherwise the heart won't start again.

When it does happen, a cardiac arrest leads to a very messy

scene. Again, you don't see it in TV dramas, but every bodily fluid is involved – blood, saliva, vomit, urine, faeces – and it takes cool, clear heads to work effectively together for the benefit of the patient. My training and experience had taught me not to panic in those circumstances but to switch into a fast-thought, calm but quick and effective mode of working. It seemed almost as if things were happening in slow motion, yet we were operating at desperate speed, because time was absolutely of the essence. Martha lay there, her staring eyes wide open, with no pulse and no rise and fall of her chest. At that moment she was effectively dead. People who have died go a strange yellowy-grey colour, but patients who have had a cardiac arrest are an intermediate colour, halfway between that and normal skin tone.

Patients who have made a Do Not Resuscitate request, or who are suffering from a terminal illness like an inoperable cancer, in which an attempt to resuscitate them would be inappropriate, have 'DNR' or 'DNAR' (Do Not Attempt Resuscitation) marked on their chart on the end of their hospital bed. This will have been discussed with the patient and next of kin. In every other case, compressions begin as soon as an arresting patient is without a pulse. However, if we catch a patient in the first moments of cardiac arrest, we can give them a 'precordial thump' – a big bash with the bottom of your clenched fist right on the sternum. The first time I did that was when working as a houseman on a renal ward; it worked, and the patient started breathing again. It's such a violent action that there is often some collateral damage, especially in elderly patients: a precordial thump is often accompanied by a crunching sound as some ribs or rib cartilage crack. But better that than a dead patient.

The moment had already passed for that to be effective in Martha's case and there was a frenzy of activity as the nurses pulled her bed away from the wall and took off the metal headboard, dropping it with a clang. We now had easy access to her from all sides. We continued compressions as a nurse brought the defibrillator and another ran in with the trolley of syringes, pre-loaded with adrenaline and atropine (which increases the heart rate) in bright yellow and green boxes. There was a tearing sound as she ripped off the cardboard wrapping.

In this, as in all cardiac arrests, we followed a predefined sequence of actions. Compressions are often enough to restart the patient's heart without the need for breathing resuscitation. If compressions do not work, the next step is to use the defibrillator. Just as in the movies, I called 'Clear!' and made sure that no one was touching the patient or the metal frame of the bed before pressing the paddles to Martha's chest. Her body jerked as the current surged through her, but her pulse did not restart. Following standard procedure, I shocked her with the paddles twice more, and resumed compressions. When she still did not resuscitate, the next step was to administer shots of adrenaline and atropine in what proved another unavailing attempt to restart Martha's heart. We had now almost run out of options. We continued with the compressions, but unfortunately, although we spent forty-five minutes battling desperately to save her, we eventually had to admit defeat and pronounce Martha dead without her ever having recovered consciousness. It was not something that was easy for any of us to accept.

During the time we had been fighting to save her life, one of the nurses had phoned Martha's family – her husband and teenage children – and said to them, 'Can you please come into the hospital at once, because she is very unwell.' Although it is important to try to make the family aware that there is an emergency, which prepares them a little for the terrible news you may have to impart, there is also a worry that if you do so over the phone, people will then be so distressed and distracted that they may have a crash or come to some other harm on their way to hospital.

I emerged from the treatment room feeling extremely disheartened and upset that we hadn't managed to bring Martha back. I could tell that all the nursing staff had the same horrible, raw feeling. As medical professionals we are there to help people; to intellectualize their health problems and find solutions to them. We make them better if we can and ease their suffering if we can't. So it was just a desperate moment because in this case there wasn't anything more we could have done.

I was now trying to prepare myself to speak to her husband and her family. Like all junior doctors, as part of my training I had been taught to break bad news in the right environment, using the right words and, since 80 per cent of communication is non-verbal, with the right posture as well. The breaking of bad news is known to be more processable by the recipient, and the response more favourable, if some form of words is first used to signal that bad news is coming. So we were trained first to give a verbal 'warning shot' such as 'I'm afraid I have some bad news for you', followed by a pause to allow them to process that information, before going on to tell them of the loss of their loved one. I was quite clear in my own mind about how I wanted to do it, but I had no time or opportunity to do so because they all suddenly appeared right in front of me. Martha's husband was standing almost nose to nose with me in the middle of the corridor, and he kept repeating, 'What is it? What is it?' And then, before I could reply, he said, 'Martha's dead, isn't she?'

'Come and talk in the office,' I said.

There were no soft words, no techniques, nothing that would help him to come to terms with what had just happened. I simply had to tell him the straight, unvarnished truth. Obviously he was distraught, and in those horrific circumstances it was very difficult to provide even an iota of comfort. That experience – the first time I had to tell someone of their partner's death – drove me to seek further training in communication with patients and their relatives at difficult times, but I discovered that, although there were several courses and advanced courses, they were all focused on breaking the news about a tumour diagnosis or something similar, not death. In the 1990s and even today, no matter how carefully the 'bad-news giver' prepares the ground in advance, telling a relative about a sudden death is extremely difficult.

Doctors working in cancer care are now automatically sent on a three-day course in advanced communication skills. When that scheme was introduced, some of those who already had an abundance of training and experience might have been a little piqued at having to undergo further training, but it is, and always has been, fundamental to the role. I value the training highly, but I remain hauntingly aware that no amount of tutelage will ever make it any easier to tell a patient that they have an inoperable cancer, or a family member that their husband, wife, mother, father, son or daughter has passed away.

Terrible things do happen without warning and it's very difficult to cushion the blow in such circumstances, but you can't help but take it a bit personally somehow as well, because the patient is under our team's care when it happens. Even worse, when you dial back and think 'How are we going to prevent that from happening in the future?' you can't really come up with an answer, because it really is just one of those awful things.

One of the most famous sayings in our world is that good surgeons know how to operate, better ones when to operate, and the best when not to operate at all. Aspiring surgeons spend upwards of ten years being taught how to perform operations, and then the next five years learning when not to. That's a very hard thing to get right because as a surgeon your instinct is always to be a very proactive, practical person. You want to use the technical skills and gifts you've developed in your years of training to solve a problem that needs fixing for a patient right then and there, and right in front of them if they are not unconscious under a general anaesthetic. It was and still is a joyous feeling to be able to do so, and an extremely privileged position to be in.

Like most medical students, I had begun my training in the belief that doctors could find a solution to any health issue, but all of us eventually have to come to the realization that some problems simply cannot be solved. Some patients also get better on their own while we are still trying to work out what is wrong with them; I often quip to my patients that my job is to make them better, or at least not make them worse, and where possible always claim the credit for their recovery. There comes a point where continued attempts to treat a patient by medical or surgical means are, sometimes literally, just prolonging the agony. One of the things we must learn – and it's a very painful lesson – is when to accept that, and step back. However, dealing with death and dying is never easy and there is an understandable temptation to delay the acceptance of the inevitable. That is only eroded with reluctance and after long experience.

I recall one woman, Jennifer, who was brought into A & E in Glasgow in considerable pain. She had been suffering from multiple sclerosis for a long time but there was now something wrong with her abdomen, and although there was no clear diagnosis, she was obviously very unwell. She was duly admitted and taken to the ward and I went to see her with the consultant, assuming that we would be able to help her. I still thought then that we could do something for everyone. We were doctors after all; we fixed things for people.

Jennifer was in a side-room with her family but they went and sat outside while we examined her. As I pulled back the bed covers I could see that her skin was purple and mottled from above her navel all the way down her legs. The consultant looked at her for a moment and then motioned for me to replace the covers. He stepped away from her bedside and lowered his voice. 'I'm afraid she isn't going to survive,' he said. 'There's been a vascular catastrophe in her abdomen, an aneurysm or something similar, and given her general health, and the effects of her MS, sadly there's nothing more to be done for her.'

He broke the sad news to Jennifer, then took her husband to one side to tell him. Other doctors might have attempted to prolong her life with a series of invasive procedures, at the price of continued pain and suffering for the patient and continued desperate anxiety for her family, until the same tragic ending was reached. So the consultant was undoubtedly right to reach the swift conclusion that nothing would be gained by further treatment, that it would do her no good and might only raise false hopes both in her and the members of her family. Better by far, surely, to tell her and her family the hard truth, manage her pain, and give them a little time to say their farewells to each other in a calm and peaceful atmosphere. In the event they had only a very short time to do so, because she died that afternoon – at long last released from her multiple sclerosis.

I was then involved in the process of producing the death certificate for her. Her body was to be cremated, and when that is to happen after a patient's death in hospital a form has to be completed, partly filled in by a junior doctor and partly by a senior one. We were always paid for completing those forms, and in the late 1990s to a young man on a relatively modest junior doctor's salary it was quite a handsome sum – from memory, £40 or £50. However, even though I was perennially short of money, I never spent those fees on food or drink or any of the usual things. Instead I always used the money to buy something that would last and that would trigger a memory of the person whose demise had brought me that modest windfall.

On this occasion I went to Waterstones in Glasgow and bought a book on Michelangelo's *Pietà*, which depicts the body of Jesus sprawled across Mary's lap after the crucifixion. I've always been a great fan of Renaissance art and of Michelangelo in particular, because of the beauty of his work and the accuracy of his depiction of human anatomy, and the *Pietà* is a beautiful statue, a perfect, enduring rendition of flesh and fabric in carved stone. I wrote Jennifer's initials and 'RIP' inside the book, and it is still on my shelves today. I have a number of other books, acquired under similarly tragic circumstances and similarly dedicated, each one a reminder of a patient we were sadly unable to save.

As well as my grounding in general surgery, there was no shortage of facial trauma for a trainee surgeon to deal with in Glasgow, and by the time I had finished my surgical training there I had seen five times as many cases as an equivalent surgical trainee would have done in London. I reached a total of 200 lower jaw fractures within two years and I wondered how many more I needed to perform to be deemed competent, but the only advice I ever received from my seniors was 'Just keep doing them, son.'

Interestingly, those undergoing surgical training in Glasgow today will see considerably fewer cases, because in Scotland over the last few years there has been a sustained 25 per cent reduction in low-energy trauma. In other words, people getting a kicking or beating is happening 25 per cent less often now than it did several years ago, although it's difficult to analyse why that is, or draw any reliable conclusions from it.

Not all low-energy trauma is the result of assault, of course. I had a case where the best man at a Glaswegian wedding came in for treatment of facial injuries after falling off a ledge at the hotel where the reception was being held. When I asked him what had happened, he said, 'Well, doctor, you know how it's the best man's duty to shag the bridesmaids? I was doing that with one of them when her husband started banging on the door. So I climbed out of the window to dodge him and slipped off the ledge.'

While I was working there, we also treated a thirteen-year-old boy who'd had a terrible accident at a cooperage in a district of Glasgow that was famously one of the most grim and notorious areas in Scotland. The accident was no less horrific for being entirely self-inflicted. The boy and his friend had sneaked into the cooperage and had been tossing burning strips of paper into a number of old vapour-filled barrels they had found lying around the place. The barrels had previously contained whisky or various chemicals and other industrial products, and to the boys' delight, the vapours in many of them were sufficiently volatile to explode with a loud 'pop' when ignited with a match. However, one barrel contained such a dangerous substance that when the boy dropped a burning taper into it, it exploded with so much force that it blew the barrel apart and blasted off the front of his face. It was so badly damaged that no reconstruction was possible using the remaining facial tissues. There was just too much of his face missing.

So as a first step we took him into the operating theatre, secured his airway and did a tracheostomy, and then attached an external fixator, an old-fashioned scaffold held in place by metal rods to keep together the remaining structures of his face – what was left of his jaw, nose and cheekbones. We cleaned out all the bits, dressed the wounds, and then transferred him to the High Dependency Unit.

We returned later to assess his injuries, once they had settled down a little bit. By the time I came back, the boy's family had turned up. His father was there, evidently drunk, and from his unkempt, dishevelled appearance and the all-too-visible signs of alcoholic excess on his face, that was clearly not an unusual occurrence. Weirdly, he seemed to find his son's tragedy highly amusing, chuckling away to himself and telling the boy, 'You're a fecking eejit, you know that?'

I did have to wonder how much parenting had been going on in that family and in such circumstances whether it would in fact be correct to say that the boy's accident was entirely his own fault.

His face was eventually reconstructed after a series of operations using sections of bone and flaps from his legs, and ultimately his appearance was restored very close to its former state. Whether that harsh lesson was enough to set him on a different, better path in life I never discovered. I hope so.

8

AFTER COMPLETING MY time as a junior houseman I became a senior houseman at Glasgow Royal Infirmary, where I began my basic training rotation: first orthopaedics, then general surgery, and then cardio-thoracic surgery. Like all junior doctors in that era, I worked punishing hours. We were on twelve-hour shifts but were also on call overnight and at weekends, and the long hours and relentless pressure we all faced could impact not just on us but on our patients too. In the rare intervals when things were quiet, the on-call doctor could crawl into a single bed squeezed into a cupboard just off the Cardiac Intensive Therapy Unit and try to grab an hour's sleep. But there was continual activity in and noise from the CITU so it was very difficult to get any rest at all, and whenever a fresh emergency cropped up my pager would start buzzing and I'd have to stagger back to work again. I was haggard, permanently exhausted, and at times would have willingly swapped all my worldly goods for a few nights of uninterrupted sleep.

Prolonged, chronic sleep deprivation is really not good for body and soul. It can lead to de-personalization (in which you feel detached from your mind and body, as if you were an outside observer of yourself) and de-realization (an alteration in how you perceive the external world, making it seem less real). My abiding memory of that period in my life is just a constant feeling of greyness; I was grey of face, grey of mind, and the world as a whole seemed a drab and colourless place.

It was the very early hours of one Monday morning in August 1999 and I'd already been awake for most of Friday, Saturday and Sunday. I'd been on call on Saturday night after doing a full shift through the day, and I had not managed a wink of sleep as a succession of emergency issues in the ITU (Intensive Treatment Unit) had my pager going off like a faulty burglar alarm. Sunday was no better, so by two o'clock on the Monday morning I had been awake non-stop for over twenty-four hours, and for most of the previous forty-eight as well. At that point we received word that, following a car crash, a patient had been taken to Intensive Care at another hospital, suffering from a devastating brain injury. Brain death had now been pronounced, and as the patient's heart was confirmed to be viable and functioning, with the permission of the next of kin it was made available to the cardio-thoracic unit for transplant.

My exhaustion was now briefly forgotten. The chance to be part of a heart transplant procedure did not come round every day.

Two candidates to receive the transplant, men with chronic heart disease and minimal life expectancy without a new heart, were immediately called in and subjected to a battery of blood tests, at the end of which the closest match to the donor, a patient called Harold, was wheeled into the operating theatre. I tried not to imagine how the loser in that particular lottery must have felt at that moment. Like prisoners on Death Row, those waiting for heart transplants can hear the clock ticking down for them and know that their time is limited. If they don't receive a new heart, they will die, sooner rather than later. So to be called into the hospital for assessment because a donor heart has been found and then to be told that someone else has the winning ticket – that another patient has proved to be a more suitable match and will be getting a new lease of life – must be absolutely devastating. Barring another heart rapidly becoming available, it is effectively close to a sentence of death.

As they awaited the results of the tests, our two patients had seemed resigned to their fates, though full of anxiety about the consequences, whichever way the dice fell for them. But I can still vividly recall the expressions on the faces of their families, particularly the wife of the man who did get the heart in the end. In her face you could read hope but also fear and deep foreboding about what was to come. Psychological distress is often worse for the partner and can impact back on the patient.

The chosen patient, Harold, was allowed a few brief moments with his wife and his family, and was then brought into the theatre suite, anaesthetized and put on to the operating table. I was scheduled to assist with the procedure, and even though I was hugely sleep-deprived, it was not a chance I was ever going to miss.

While we were setting up the operation, the donor heart was removed from the dead crash victim in the hospital where his body had been taken after the accident by the retrieval team. It was placed in a temperature-controlled polyurethane container and couriered to Glasgow by helicopter – a flight taking only a few minutes – then rushed down to the operating theatre, where it was transferred to a green plastic receptacle that reminded me a bit of the Tupperware bowls in my mother's kitchen.

The consultant who would be carrying out the procedure had donned a pair of operating loupes with three and a half times magnification. Those telescope-like lenses projecting from his eyes while he was operating made him look less like a surgeon than something out of *Doctor Who*. He was a very skilful surgeon with gifted, quick fingers – when he was tying knots in sutures, for example – and I was in awe of the pace and precision with which he worked. If his patients had been aware of it they would have been in awe of it too, because that speed of hand was very good news for them: the less time patients spend under general anaesthetic, the quicker their recovery.

The heart was just sitting there in the green plastic bowl. The scrub nurse was standing next to it and completely ignoring it as she got on with her own preparations, but I couldn't resist taking a look at it. The bowl was filled with a clear, glassy-looking saline solution, and in the bottom of it, shining in the glow of the operating theatre lights, was this brownish-red object the size of a medium-sized clenched fist, with tubes and pipes – arteries and veins – protruding from it. It was hard to equate that insignificant-looking object with its role as the giver of life – even harder, in some ways, to imagine it happily beating away in the chest of the donor just hours before – but if everything went to plan it would soon be the source of a near-miraculous transformation, turning the unconscious, desperately ill body lying on the operating table in front of me back into a functioning human being again.

The bright lights illuminating the operating table cast the rest of the room into relative darkness, increasing the drama of the scene as the consultant began the procedure by opening Harold's chest from the bottom of his neck to the top of his abdomen. After peeling back the flesh, he then cut through the breastbone with an electric saw. Harold had been suffering from ischaemic heart disease, so he had had previous problems with blocked arteries that had already led to several heart attacks. He had also had chest surgery for a coronary by-pass, and the stainless steel wires used to secure his breastbone after that operation were still in place and had to be removed again. His healed breastbone and the two halves of his chest were then re-separated along the mid-line.

The electric saw, always used downwards from the neck towards the abdomen to avoid any possibility of the blade slipping and cutting the patient's chin, made a powerful rumbling whine and the grinding noise of the saw-blade on bone seemed shockingly loud in the cloistral hush of the operating theatre. The heat it generated also caused a smell like burning hair as the collagen in the bone heated and burned, and a fine mist of tiny bone fragments was thrown up, glittering like frost particles under the brilliant theatre lights.

We used retractors to pull the ribs back, opening up the chest cavity and exposing the heart. I had to exert some firm pressure to wind the retractors apart, and as I did so I could hear the creaking, crunching and cracking sounds as Harold's ribs were forced apart, and felt the vibrations transmitted through his chest to my scrubbed and gloved hands and forearms. There was one immediate complication: the previous surgery Harold had undergone had caused the front wall of his heart to become stuck to the back wall of his thorax – effectively the ribs – so the consultant had to carefully separate that before he could continue the operation. While he was doing that, I just had to stand still, holding the retractors on the other side of the patient, and trying to shake off my fatigue.

All of a sudden there was a *whoosh* and blood began spurting from Harold's heart. There's an old saying in surgery that you only worry about bleeding when you can hear it, and I could definitely hear this, because gouts of blood were cascading from Harold's chest on to the operating table and then splashing down on to the floor.

Part of the heart muscle is severely damaged in a heart attack and the wall of the heart then repairs with a thin layer of fibrous scar tissue that doesn't expand and contract and can form an aneurysm (a swelling) of the heart wall. There had been just such a defect in Harold's heart, formed after one of his earlier heart attacks, and while separating the heart wall from the thorax, the surgeon had inadvertently opened a hole through this weakened area into the left ventricle. As a result, with every beat of Harold's heart, blood at a pressure of 120 millimetres of mercury was spurting out of the ventricle on to the floor.

The consultant gave a little cry of surprise and then said to me, 'Quickly, put your hand in there!'

At once, I squeezed my hand past the cut edge of the sternum, into the chest cavity. Even through my surgical glove I could feel the warmth of the blood bathing my hand and the ragged pumping of Harold's heart, but as I balled my hand into a fist and pressed it against the hole in his heart, the blood flow began to slow. The pressure of my hand was now all that was stopping the beating of his heart from expelling his entire blood volume. The heart pushes out 70 to 90 millilitres of blood with every beat and the body only contains about six litres to start with, so it wouldn't have taken very long for the whole lot to go down the drain, and losing even 40 per cent of your blood is life-threatening.

While I stood there like the fabled Dutch boy with his finger in the dyke, instead of opening up the big blood vessels next to the heart the consultant rapidly switched to Harold's groin and started opening the femoral vessels there so he could connect the heart by-pass machine using those. Even with his quick, sure hands it still took him several minutes to get on to the vessels, isolate them and place cannulas in them. All the while I had to stand very still beside the patient with my left arm buried up to the wrist in his chest and my hand deep in his heart, bathed by the warm, slippery blood that was also soaking my surgical gown and turning it steadily more crimson.

I watched the unfolding fight for Harold's life through the surgical letterbox-shape formed between the mask over my mouth and nose, and the cap covering my hair, leaving just the narrow strip around my eyes exposed. I was conscious of every sensation: the roughish, slightly starchy feel of my surgical scrubs, the antiseptic smell, and the constant faint, slightly metallic tang of blood in my nostrils.

You would have thought that the adrenaline rush as we battled to save this patient's life would have made even a sloth sit up and pay attention. Yet despite the sheer drama of what was going on in front of me, I was so sleep-deprived that, standing motionless in that very hot atmosphere, listening to the hypnotic *bleep . . . bleep . . . bleep* of the anaesthetic machine, I fell into a micro-sleep. I just dropped off with my hand still inside Harold's chest.

I jerked awake again an instant later, wondering where I was. Then the realization dawned. Fortunately, even though I had slept for a fraction of a second, I hadn't released the pressure of my fist on Harold's heart, so blood was still only seeping rather than pumping from it. I cast a surreptitious look around the operating table to see if anyone else had noticed what had happened, then dug my fingernails into the palm of my free hand and opened my eyes as wide as I could, determined to force myself to stay awake and alert. Yet, astonishingly, I soon found myself jerking awake after another micro-sleep, and whatever I did it continued to happen, multiple times. I simply couldn't control it. Each time I thought, 'Jesus! Come on, Jim, you've got to stay awake!' But I was so exhausted that I'd only last a few more seconds and then drop off again. Yet at some subconscious level, even while I was dropping off to sleep I must have known that I had to maintain the pressure on his left ventricle, and I'd find myself snapping back to wakefulness after yet another micro-sleep still with my hand holding back the floodtide of blood – Harold's life essence.

Once the consultant succeeded in connecting the femoral artery to the by-pass machine, the immediate crisis was past. He then moved back to the right side of Harold's chest, facing me across the operating table, and readied him for the process called cold cardioplegia – the means by which we stop the heart beating before removing it. The heart cavity was opened up and then flooded with iced, sterilized potassium solution, which stopped the native heart dead. The veins and arteries to it were clamped, yet, even though his own heart was no longer beating, the gleaming by-pass machine continued the heart's functions, circulating blood and oxygen around Harold's body and keeping him alive.

With the native heart no longer trying to expel his lifeblood, I was finally able to release the pressure on the hole in Harold's heart and withdraw my hand. My arm had been stuck in the same position for so long that it was agonizing to move it but I stifled a yelp of pain, reminding myself that the patient in front of me had rather worse problems to deal with than an attack of cramp in his hand.

I then assisted the consultant as he began to sever the arteries and veins, ready for the removal of the heart, the core of Harold's being. For some bizarre reason it made me think of the Aztecs, even though they didn't remove the hearts of their sacrificial victims by breaking the ribs apart but instead by stabbing up through the abdomen and diaphragm, and then just pulling the heart down through the diaphragm and out through the abdominal wall.

Before removing the heart, the consultant carefully separated the back wall and left it in place as a secure site for attaching the donor heart. It would then be in the perfect position to connect to the aorta and the other great vessels of the heart. He then removed the remainder of the old and damaged heart which, like any other surplus tissue removed during an operation, was simply tossed into a container with the swabs and other surgical waste, ready for disposal by fire in the hospital's furnaces. Even though it was badly damaged and defective, it still seemed almost shocking to think of a human heart being treated in that way.

Harold was now lying on the operating table with his chest open and his heart removed – a hollow shell – and when all was in readiness we lifted the donor heart out of its saline bath and inserted it in the chest cavity. The consultant first attached it to the back wall of the native heart and then began connecting all the veins and arteries. Once more I was in awe of the speed at which he worked, his fingers seeming to fly as he carried out the suturing. He was moving almost too fast to follow yet every stitch was absolutely precise and calculated.

At the end of the procedure, when the operation was almost complete, he restarted Harold's new heart with two paddles. In one sense it was a familiar, almost clichéd scene, repeated in a thousand hospital dramas on TV: the medic holding two paddles against the patient's chest, calling 'Clear!' to make sure that none of the medical staff is touching the patient, and then the convulsive jerk of the patient's body as electric current surges through his chest, restarting the heart. The difference in this case was that this was no fictional drama and the paddles were not resting on the patient's chest but were actually touching the heart itself. Once again it was an astonishing thing to see the heart, lifeless one moment, reanimate the next and begin to beat, and slowly settle into a steady rhythm. It felt as if I was witness to a miracle.

The by-pass machine was disconnected and wheeled away and we began to close, inserting drains and removing the retractors that had been holding back the ribs. We bound together the severed halves of the sternum with a new length of stainless steel wire, and finally we sutured the livid scar line running from Harold's neck to his abdomen. Once he had been transferred to the Intensive Care Unit and all his vital signs had been reported as OK, there were handshakes all round and a feeling of huge elation at the success of the operation. But in my case that soon gave way to yet more waves of crushing tiredness.

By the time we finished it was about six in the morning and I fell into bed absolutely exhausted; but I had to be up again within a couple of hours, ready to accompany the consultant to see Harold at eight o'clock. When we entered the ICU, we were greeted by a stunning sight. The night before he'd been lying on the operating table with his chest open and his heart removed, an empty shell maintained by a machine and looking like a corpse. That had been amazing enough, but it was even more stupefying to see the same man a few hours later, waking up and opening his eyes – almost resurrected, a revitalized, sentient human being once more.

When I reflected on the operation afterwards, I was not merely running through the stages of the procedure in my mind, filing away every detail for future reference, against the day when I would be leading a surgical team of my own. I was also offering a silent prayer of thanks that my series of micro-sleeps during the most critical phase of the procedure had not had any damaging consequences.

The term 'acquired psychopathy' is sometimes applied to the state the sleep-deprived surgical trainees of yesteryear could find themselves in, and it might even have been considered to be beneficial in surgical circles, because the blunting of young surgeons' senses and feelings might help them to carry out surgical procedures without the distractions of empathy or compassion for the patient. I felt at the time, and continue to believe, that this was a dangerous and possibly mythical idea. The fact that the sleep deprivation imposed on junior doctors in the past indubitably had serious consequences, including my falling asleep during a heart transplant procedure, has always seemed to me to be a demonstrable failure of modern medicine that should have been addressed long before it was.

In the UK, the campaign to reduce the exhausting, crazy hours junior doctors were expected to work ultimately proved successful, but as I write, the government is seeking to reverse that hard-won protection for doctors and patients alike. I am horror-struck at the thought because there is absolutely no question that tired doctors can make mistakes and tired doctors can fall asleep – even when one of their fists is blocking a hole in a patient's heart to stop his lifeblood spilling on to the floor. The mistakes that tired doctors make might even kill their patients.

There may be a financial cost in restricting the hours junior doctors work but there may also be a terrible human cost in extending them. On the occasion I've just described I was lucky: Harold survived, mainly thanks to the skill of the consultant operating on him, but partly also because of the sheer good fortune that my micro-sleeps did not have fatal results. But if we are to avert needless tragedies in the future, those over-long hours for doctors have to be a thing of the past, not the present or future.

9

AS THE NEW millennium unfolded I was now beginning to carry out proper facial surgery and assisting at major cancer operations. I was allowed to do the close on arms after flaps had been raised from them, and I was actually treating some skin cancers and facial traumas, and looking after patients with serious infections.

The first time I raised a flap to reconstruct the face myself, I was told to take it from a patient's forearm. I was pretty nervous about it because a lot can go wrong when taking a flap from there, including damaging the motor nerves and muscles. You also have to anticipate where the important blood vessels will be, and it does vary quite considerably between individuals. In someone who has a physical job, or works out a lot, the muscle will have grown around the blood vessels, whereas a sedentary old person's blood vessels will just meander in between the muscle layers.

I had been revising the anatomy the night before and was still doing so the following morning as I got ready to go to the theatre suite. Even when I knew the anatomy backwards, I still tended to walk into the theatre suite with a reference book – a sort of atlas on how to go about these things – under my arm, using it as a kind of lucky charm.

On that first time raising a flap, the consultant supervising me, Stuart Hislop, did his best to put me at my ease, saying,

'You've got two hours, Jim, so there's plenty of time. I'm here if you need me, but just take your time.' I was reassured that he had confidence in me and believed I wouldn't make a mess of it, and I knew that I could ask for his help if I needed it, so I got the tourniquet on the arm and cracked on with it. I managed to do it, and did it well, though I used every minute of those two hours, working slowly and carefully to make sure I got it right. These days I can do the same procedure in about twenty-five minutes.

The aim in surgery is obviously always to avoid mistakes and to maintain your concentration throughout, because a moment's inattention can have potentially fatal consequences. So far in my surgical career I've avoided any disastrous errors, but towards the end of my surgical training there was a moment when I went on to autopilot, though luckily the only consequence was that we went for lunch a couple of hours later than normal.

As a surgical trainee, normally you'd dissect a flap ready for transplant but then leave it attached to the blood supply while removing the tumour with the other surgeon. Normally we'd all then have a break and come back in afterwards to complete the operation. However, on this occasion, having finished the preparation of the flap, I carried straight on and cut across the radial artery, severing the blood flow to the flap. I realized at once what I'd done, and experienced a sinking feeling, but plucking up my courage, I said to the consultant, 'Erm, Stuart, would it be OK if we pressed on and inset the flap and did the micro first and then had lunch afterwards?'

He looked at me across the operating table – luckily my blushes were mostly hidden by the surgical mask – and replied, 'Why?'

There was no hiding place now. 'Because I've just ligated the radial artery.'

Some consultants would have exploded at that point, but he was calm about it. 'Ahhh,' he said. 'OK, we'll have lunch a wee bit later today.' And we completed the operation and then went for a bite to eat.

Not long afterwards I was raising the arm flap with another trainee and after two hours the tourniquet was squashing the arm and the volume had to be let down to prevent tissue damage. You have to warn the anaesthesia team when you're going to release the tourniquet because, having been without blood and oxygen, that part of the body will flood the circulation with metabolites (the products of metabolic reactions), causing the blood pressure to drop.

So we told the anaesthetists and then let the tourniquet down, but it turned out that I had inadvertently damaged a side-branch on an artery. Blood was pouring out, and I could tell it was arterial because it was a vivid red colour and it rushed out in bright rivulets, unlike darker, venous blood which oozes more slowly from an arm.

The consultant looked at me and said, 'OK, over to you.'

I thought, 'Shit, what have I damaged here?' At first I reckoned it was the main brachial artery, supplying the whole arm. This worried me and I could feel myself going hot and cold, while the room seemed unusually bright, and for a moment I was once again that nervous medical student who had fainted at his first sight of an operation in progress. But then I took a deep breath, focused on the problem and got straight to work. The first step was to stop it bleeding, so I put a finger on it to stem it, got a vascular stitch from the nurse, sutured across the artery and stopped the flow. In the event it was not the brachial artery but a smaller one – a tributary, rather than the main river, if you like – and everything turned out OK in the end.

I was in a similar situation with a trainee recently, with a patient who'd previously had radiotherapy and had a very fibrosed neck. When the trainee put the clamps on the internal jugular vein, the blood flow just wouldn't stop. Blood was pouring past the clamp, and she looked at me and said, 'What do I do now?'

I reached across, put some pressure on it with my finger and said, 'The first thing to do is to stop it bleeding, and then that gives us some thinking time.'

The clamps are only just strong enough to stop the blood flow in a normal healthy patient and are not made any stronger because we don't want them damaging the blood vessel. In this case, the fibrous tissue in the patient's neck was tough enough to hold the clamp open, so we just needed to get a slightly stronger clamp and use that instead. The experience of having been a trainee yourself in the past and having those moments of panic when you see rivulets of arterial blood pouring out fast not only makes you sympathetic to what your trainee is going through in similar circumstances, it also teaches you that there's always a solution. Just using your finger to stem the flow while you take a moment to think about things will enable you to come up with the right one.

Being aware of the bigger picture is important too. Early on in my surgical career we had to treat the victim of a horrific traffic accident who had multiple injuries. The orthopaedic surgeon, an enthusiastic senior registrar, was busily opening up the bilateral lower-leg tibia and fibula fractures and cutting into the fascia to ease the pressure within the muscles that was decreasing blood flow and preventing blood and oxygen from reaching the nerve and muscle cells. However, at the other end of the operating table the patient was so close to dying that eventually the anaesthetist had to say, 'You need to stop what you're doing now, because this patient is not going to survive it.'

The registrar bristled, and said, 'I've never been asked to do that before.'

'Maybe, but I'm telling you that if you carry on, the patient will not survive.'

Even though in other circumstances it would have been the correct surgical procedure, in this case the patient's other injuries were so serious that he was unlikely to survive them anyway, and certainly would not have done had he had to undergo the surgery and blood loss necessary to repair his shattered legs. If he survived, his leg injuries could be treated at a later stage; if not, he deserved to be allowed as dignified a death as possible, without undergoing pointless surgery.

After finishing my time as a senior house officer, I was in competition with everyone else who had reached the same stage to get a 'training number' and become a registrar in a speciality. In a smallish speciality where there are only 300 or so consultant posts there is always a bit of a waxing and waning in the number available. I was applying to be a specialist registrar at Canniesburn Hospital in Bearsden, Glasgow, which enjoyed a reputation as the best maxillofacial department in Scotland, but a couple of people had recently been appointed to the rotation there, so that left just one available job and twelve candidates chasing it. Most of the senior staff I'd been working with were very supportive when they heard I'd applied, but one consultant just sucked his teeth for a moment, then said, 'Well, it's a very strong field,' in a tone that suggested he thought I'd have more chance of being struck by lightning than being chosen.

So I said to him, 'Well, do you know my view of it? It's like a swimming race: you acknowledge that there are other people present in the other lanes but I plan to touch the wall first.' That was truly what I thought. Whatever ambitions you have, there are always going to be pretty good people around, so what are you going to do? Just throw the towel in and say, 'Why don't you give it to one of those other eleven talented people and I'll just give up now'?

So I persevered. I was in an Italian restaurant over the road from where the interview had taken place, having met Lorna and the kids there either for a celebration or a drowning of the sorrows, depending on the result, when the senior consultant phoned me and told me I had got the job.

Canniesburn was a plastic and jaw unit set up on the Harold Gillies model. It could be a bit of a nightmare to work there because, even though people were having major facial surgery, there was no overnight anaesthetic cover, so if the airway on a patient was threatened during the night, by bleeding or swelling after the operation, the only option was to put them in an ambulance and send them down the road, sirens blaring, blue lights flashing, and hope they got to the next hospital in time. So there was a lot of risk, and in fact the hospital was closed down during my second year there and I spent the remainder of my time as a specialist registrar at the Southern General in Linthouse, Glasgow – or 'Suffering Genitals' as it was irreverently known by junior doctors.

A year into my job as a specialist registrar I was awarded a clinical research fellowship at the Beatson Laboratories in Bearsden, and for the next four years I worked part-time in the labs and part-time in the clinical unit. I joined Ken Parkinson's research group which was looking into targeting telomeres at the ends of chromosomes, which are vulnerable in cancer cells. There are twenty-three pairs of chromosomes in each cell. Cancer develops from one of them going wrong and then forms a whole clone – a bunch of bad cells that damage your body and, if they are not completely eradicated, will eventually kill you. By the time the cancer is detectable, the cancerous lump will be formed of about a billion cells in one cubic centimetre; if it grows to a trillion cells, it is not survivable. We recently reclassified staging for head and neck cancer following evidence that the bigger a tumour, the lower the survival chances. Put bluntly, size does matter.

Whenever a human cell replicates, it produces a slightly shorter chromosome with each copy and eventually there is no more material left and the cell ceases to replicate. It's a natural part of the ageing process and the reason why we are all fated to die in the end. However, cancer cells copy themselves many thousands of times over and get round this obstacle by reactivating a specific enzyme. The research I did at the Beatson showed that if you damage the enzyme used by the cancer cells, it makes them much more sensitive to radiation than normal cells, which has obvious benefits for cancer patients undergoing radiotherapy. That was the conclusion of my thesis, part of which was published in *The Lancet Oncology* and *Cancer Research* and earned me my stripes as a research scientist.

I wanted to start as a consultant with a proper science PhD

because scientists can be sniffy about doctors – often for good reasons – and it was the only way to have a serious chance of building a research team in the clinical environment, as opposed to just doing the job. I finished my final training in 2005 and without a clinical research team I would have been facing doing the same operations, in the same way, for the rest of my career, rather than being involved in improving and enhancing the treatment I could offer.

Having completed their five-year training period, all registrars must pass an exam before graduating to a consultant's role. It was an oral and clinical exam only when I took it: we examined a series of patients and then answered questions to test our knowledge of their conditions and were grilled by senior consultants. Not long before that time, surgeons had imagined that this exam would be more like a 'fireside chat' than a serious test after finishing training – mainly because they were told so! However, the final surgical exam had evolved by the time I got there and it rapidly became evident that it was much more intense than that – a fact emphasized when some people failed it.

Even when I'd cleared that hurdle I still needed to demonstrate that I had done enough hours in the operating theatre and had enough cases in my surgical log-book to progress to the next stage. That had to be signed off by a specialist advisory committee, whereupon I was finally given my Completion of Training Certificate. But even though I was now qualified to be a consultant, it was not an automatic process: no one actually becomes a consultant until they have found a hospital willing to employ them. The Regional Unit at the Southern General Hospital in Glasgow and then afterwards the Dumfries and Galloway Royal Infirmary duly offered me locum posts, so after spending almost twenty years in dental, medical and surgical training, I had finally become a consultant.

After eight months of this work in Glasgow and Dumfries, in 2006 I became Consultant Surgeon at the Bradford Teaching Hospitals in West Yorkshire, and the work I did there and the clinical trials I supervised over the next eight years brought me to the attention of the Royal Marsden Hospital in London, one of the world's foremost cancer hospitals. In April 2014 I was recruited as a consultant there, and spent three years in London before returning to Glasgow, to the Queen Elizabeth University Hospital – the largest hospital in western Europe, built on the site of the old Southern General – as Consultant Surgeon in Maxillofacial/Head and Neck Surgery and head of my own clinical research team. Lorna, as a Specialist Consultant in Restorative Dentistry, often works with my team. Her career has paralleled my own.

10

SURGERY, IN ANY of the nine specialities (cardio-thoracic, oral
and maxillofacial, trauma and orthopaedic, otolaryngology –
ear, nose and throat – paediatric, plastic, urology, neurosurgery
and general surgery), requires a great deal of training and practice in order to develop the knowledge base and the necessary
diagnostic and technical skills for safe and effective clinical
work. It takes years of practice and rehearsal before a musician
is ready to play a solo concert, and if you want to fly fast jets in
the RAF you have to go through countless hours of training in
a simulator before you are unleashed on the real thing. Yet,
strangely, considering the constant stream of life-or-death decisions we have to make, surgical training is very different, because
our fine technical skills are still largely developed at the operating table, working on live patients. All surgical trainees are now
required to complete a basic skills course – the fundamentals of
suturing, wound care and management – and some specialist
courses are also available, but simulation training is still fairly
rudimentary.

I found it deeply frustrating when working at one of my previous hospitals, when I could have got a second-hand microsurgery
microscope (probably from the USA on eBay) and told my
juniors 'Go warm up on that', or 'Practise on Thursday and Friday, because you're going to be doing micro on Monday', and
that would have brought them on; but there was simply neither

the space available at the hospital nor the funds to buy the equipment, so the trainees had to continue to learn on the job, albeit always under the close supervision of myself or another consultant.

In training this way with real patients it is important to break up tasks into achievable components and set these up for the trainees, making it as straightforward as possible for them, in order to increase the chances of successful completion of the tasks and therefore help them gain confidence. Many of the trainees who have passed through my hands have gone on to become very skilled at microsurgery in their own right, and that is lovely to see. It is also very valuable to have a skilled surgeon on the other side of the microscope, and we work as a team. We concentrate for up to four hours at a time in these operations before we take a break, and while you might think that you are still as sharp as a tack at the end of that time period as you were at the beginning, it can be useful to have another pair of eyes. Just occasionally, when you have already been operating for several hours, you might hesitate for an instant and think 'This way or that way?', or you will have a tiny gap in a vein that you are suturing and you're not sure whether to use one suture or two. If you have complete confidence in the other surgeon you can just say 'Two in there or one?', and he will say 'I think one', and that resolves the momentary doubt.

Surgical assisting is also a very active, skilled process and not merely a passive holding of retractors. When training at the highest level, I have often felt when we change over, because the microsurgery problem needs me to perform it, that the trainee is assisting me a little better than I was assisting them, such is their highly developed ability to do so. When training new surgeons I often use similar techniques to teaching music (both are very high-level motor functions), one of which is 'visualization'. Through functional MRI scanning, the areas of the brain involved in complex movements have been shown to be active during the process of visualization of those same movements. So, like a gymnast visualizing a triple somersault before performing it for the first time, I ask trainee surgeons to imagine as vividly as possible that the difficult microsurgery task they are about to undertake is happening before their eyes and being performed by their fingers, because I know that the execution of a complex surgical manoeuvre immediately following such visualization will often be more successful than if they'd come to it cold.

As they become more competent and confident, we allow trainees to do parts of, and later the whole of, a procedure but, just as a trainee pilot is only allowed to do a difficult landing on a stormy day at the very end of his training, once he has mastered everything else, our trainee surgeons graduate to doing the resection of a tumour only when they are flawless at every other part of the procedure. I'm sure for the trainees, just as it was for me, when the consultant finally says 'Right, you're fine now, you do the resection', it does induce a moment of moderate panic and the thought 'Whaaat?! Are you sure?'

Even when fully trained, the surgeon's role can never be a simple, cold, calculated process of assessing a patient's symptoms, deciding on an appropriate course of treatment and then carrying it out. It is vital that we all remember, at all times, that we are not just dealing with a collection of organs, skin, flesh and bone, the diseases that attack them and the symptoms they present. We should never lose sight of the fact that we are caring for vital, sentient human beings with hopes, fears, feelings and emotional vulnerabilities that must be taken into account, and they also have close friends and family members who care deeply for them.

We hold multi-disciplinary team meetings to discuss our patients and their tumours, to establish whether we can treat them for cure, and if so, the best way to do that. Over the years I've attended scores of such meetings at hospitals in the West of Scotland, Yorkshire and London, and I've found that the best way to discuss each case is if it is accompanied by a series of PowerPoint slides projected on to a screen, so that everyone can see for themselves the location of the cancer, its appearance and spread. And I always make sure that the patient's face appears as the first slide in each presentation, and that the image is then repeated in the corner of every subsequent slide while we discuss the issues relevant to that particular case. It ensures that the professionals in the room are aware of the individual person, their extended family and their particular set of personal circumstances rather than just holding a purely clinical, almost abstract discussion about a tumour. Without that constant visual reminder of our patients' humanity, the time constraints and competitive pressures of the meeting could sometimes lead to a less compassionate discussion. So for me, the gold standard is when the patient's face is presented, and that image gives everyone an immediate insight into how kind or otherwise life appears to have been for that individual. The person whose cancer we are aiming to treat becomes an almost tangible presence in the room, and I'm sure that helps us to improve the quality of our care.

When I review cases, some of those images are of patients

whose lives we have saved or transformed, but others are haunting reminders of lives cut short, often well before their natural span.

May was a retired nurse in her late eighties, with silver hair touching her shoulders. When she came to my clinic she was in a wheelchair pushed by her granddaughter, who steered it to the side of the desk in my consulting room. May had a calm, serene countenance, and when she spoke she was measured in her words. She told me that there had been an odd-looking patch on the side of her tongue for many years and she had been cared for by a number of different surgeons. However, recently this misbehaving piece of oral mucosa (the thin layer of skin that covers the interior of body parts including the nose and mouth, and the respiratory, digestive and genito-urinary tracts, and which produces mucus to protect them) had developed into a lump and had now become a rather large mass on the side of her tongue. While not yet impairing her ability to speak clearly, this was obviously becoming a pressing issue.

I have often found that this is the most frustrating of scenarios. The locality of the lump – the mouth – is easy to see and it should be much more straightforward to discover when cells are misbehaving and turning into cancer cells which will kill a patient than, for example, in the rectum (in the case of colorectal cancer) or deep within the lung tissue, or even within the depths of normal breast tissue, when a two-millimetre deposit can turn into a sizeable tumour. Why then can we not find the indicators on such a clearly visible oral mucosa that will tell us when a previously harmless patch of tissue is about to become a life-threatening tumour and remove it before this occurs?

May had first been seen by one of my colleagues, who had organized an initial work-up including a biopsy of this new lump and some CT imaging. Encouragingly, the images showed that the new mass was entirely confined to the oral part of her tongue and had not penetrated the root where it joined the throat. As a result, although a cancer is never good news, in surgical terms it was 'very resectable' – that is to say, it would be possible to achieve a sufficient margin around the lump to remove it and effect a cure ... but not in a person of May's mature years and poor state of overall health.

When the biopsy results had been returned, I held a team meeting to discuss our approach to May's treatment, and then began to prepare to meet May. I wanted to break the news of her cancer in a very careful fashion while also respecting her past nursing experience. A clinical nursing specialist was also in the room with us, sitting alongside May, ready to offer her any emotional support she might need. As ever when I have to deliver bad news, all of my senses seemed to become hyper-acute and I was aware of all the background noises from outside my room – the murmur of conversations, the sound of passing footsteps – that would normally have passed unnoticed. I tried to shut my ears to those extraneous sounds, and the walls seemed to close in around us as I held May's eyes in what I hoped was a confident gaze, not wishing to look away.

'The results are back from your biopsy, May,' I said, then paused for a few seconds. 'And I'm afraid that it's not the best news we could have hoped for.'

I always find that the hardest part of breaking bad news is not to collapse into the chasm opening before me, the bad news messenger, and start blurting out information in an uncontrolled stream that a patient in an understandably distressed state might not be able fully to comprehend. After another pause, which lasted only a few seconds but felt absolutely interminable, I told her that the results showed that there was a new growth on her tongue. 'It is likely to get bigger and it also appears to be invading the underlying tissue.'

'Is it cancer?' she said, her voice so low I had to strain to hear her.

'Yes, I'm afraid it is, May. It's cancer.'

At this point I would normally have explained to my patient that their cancer and their experience of it was unlikely to be similar to any cancer that had affected the last person they could remember who had died of the disease. Cancers vary enormously, not just from type to type but also from individual to individual, as do the patients suffering from them, and what is an eminently curable cancer in one patient may be an inoperable sentence of death for another. However, May was a former nurse who had had many years' experience in hospitals before she eventually left the profession to run her own businesses and, as much from what she did not say as what she did, I was beginning to get the feeling that she'd had experience of patients with oral cavity cancer in the past.

'So what now?' she said.

'The multi-disciplinary team have been discussing your situation at our team meeting this morning,' I said. 'Unfortunately, given your general health and condition [her daughter had earlier told me that her mother could only walk fifty yards on level ground and could not attempt a flight of stairs], we have reached the sad conclusion that the major surgery required to remove this lump and reconstruct your tongue for function, possibly followed by radiotherapy, would be more likely to end your life than to save it.'

Once more I paused to allow her to digest those terrible

words. It was the worst possible news a human being could hear: a sentence of death upon her.

'I'm very sorry, May,' I said.

Although the concerns of the treating surgical team pale into insignificance beside those of our patient, a decision not to go ahead with a course of treatment is always an extremely difficult moment for all of us. Technically, looking at this case in purely surgical terms, we knew that we could have achieved a cure of the cancer. The balance was tipped against doing so because, in her weakened condition, the treatment to effect the cure would have ended May's life anyway.

Despite the traumatic news I was giving her, throughout our conversation up to that point May had remained sitting upright, with a generally composed expression, maintaining her dignified demeanour, but I saw that she was now silently weeping. As I looked at her, I had to fight to control the tears that were starting to prick my own eyes. The nursing specialist sitting alongside May handed her a paper tissue, held her hand and gently laid her other hand on May's shoulder, offering her some sympathy and consolation.

After allowing May enough time to recover her poise a little, I began to talk to her about how we would try to control the lump as much as possible and make sure that she was comfortable so that, if we could not cure her, we could at least ease her discomfort and manage her pain. Although at that time she was experiencing very little pain, I had to warn her that this was likely to change in the future. The lump was not yet causing her difficulty in terms of speaking or swallowing, and nor was it bleeding, but again I told her – though her experience as a nurse may already have made her aware of it – that all those things were almost certain to change and become issues in the future.

Since we had ruled out surgery as an option, although she would be seeing the nursing specialist and other medical and palliative care staff in the future, my first meeting with May would almost certainly also be my last. As we said our good-byes I wished her well, and she thanked me for my help and time, and then raised a hand in farewell as she was wheeled from the room. After she had gone the room felt very empty and somehow much bigger. I was left with the familiar hollow feeling of impotent failure and regret that we do not have some-thing better to treat these abnormally growing cells that derive from normal healthy mouth tissue.

With that long-standing pre-cancerous patch in her mouth, May fell into a category of patients that for many years I have felt we must be able to do better by. Yet, even in 2018, we are still unable to identify the exact biomarkers (the molecules in the human body that give an indication that something may or may not be happening – for example, the prostate-specific anti-gens that indicate if prostate cancer is present) or any clear signs that would tell us when a patch of mouth lining that appears abnormal is likely to turn into an aggressive tumour, and when it can be safely left alone.

One of the difficulties here is that when treating such a patch surgically, common practice in the past has been either to remove it with a laser or even vaporize it, again using a laser. The problem with lasering out the patch is that the technique removes all the tissue and therefore if no cancer develops we cannot subsequently tell how much risk of it there had actually been. By the same token, without previous tissue samples for a patient who then develops a tumour, we have no biomarkers to tell us which were the indicators for the development of that cancer. Laser vaporization of unhealthy tissue is, to me, the perfect wrong treatment. If all of the tissue is turned into smoke, we firstly don't know what was there, and secondly cannot be certain that none of it has been left behind.

All patients undergoing surgical treatment for cancer will first have been subjected to a biopsy – that is to say, a small piece of tissue will have been sampled from 'the worst appearing area' of a patch. This is placed under a microscope and then, because most cells are colourless and transparent and have to be stained in order to be visible, it is usually coloured with haematoxylin (a violet or dark blue stain) and eosin (a red stain) – the most widely used and reliable stains employed in histology. The specimen is then assessed by an expert pathologist in the same way it has been done since the invention of this technique in 1876, with the stains revealing the different constituents of the specimen under the microscope, making it easier to distinguish and identify them.

While degrees of change in the size and shape of cells and the nucleus they contain can give an indication of degree of risk, we still have no reliable way of identifying cells that will go rogue and become tumours. For a patient in a poor general state of health, whether as a result of age, general infirmity or poor lifestyle choices, the end result of our failure to identify and give effective treatment to an abnormal patch of mucosa while still at a pre-cancerous stage may be their eventual death from the subsequent cancer. While such a cancer may appear curable on a scan, for a dignified and composed but frail and elderly ex-nurse like May it became a death sentence because the treatment to cure her cancer would have ended her life anyway.

In May's case, it was clear almost from the start that we would be unable to do anything for her but offer palliative care and make her eventual passing as pain-free and peaceful as possible. Other patients with similarly bleak prospects pose very different dilemmas for us.

Kathleen was an elderly lady with a large tumour in her mouth who was brought into the hospital by members of her very supportive family. Her tongue had mostly been replaced by the tumour which was not only painful and tending to bleed but badly infected too, evidenced by the bad smell emanating from it. There was also a chaotic blood supply to the tongue – another consequence of the cancer and the way it was disrupting the body's normal functions.

The name cancer – 'the crab', as all astrologers will tell you – allegedly goes all the way back to Hippocrates in ancient Greece. It was so named because, unlike normal vascularity, cancer-supplying blood vessels have an abnormal crab-claw appearance. Cancer blood vessels are immature, and while the walls of normal, healthy, mature arteries contain a protein called actin, cancer vessels contain a protein called tubulin which makes them much less robust. This information does help us with some approaches, one example being the use of electro-chemotherapy to collapse and destroy the cancerous blood vessels without causing much damage to the normal ones.

Cancer lumps are often not well supplied with oxygen and any cell more than 150 microns (or 150 thousandths of a millimetre) from a capillary will not survive, because that is how far oxygen diffuses in tissue fluid: no oxygen, no tumour survival. As a result, you get necrosis (cell death) within the mass of the tumour, and necrotic human tissue is the best culture medium you can get for the bacteria that produce horrible smells. It is literally the stink of death, the bacterial colonization producing putrefaction and a rotten odour that evolution has taught us to get right away from because it's got bad stuff in it.

The active chemical, ethyl mercaptan, is allegedly detectable by humans in concentrations as low as 0.36 parts per billion. Vultures can pick it up in even more minute concentrations. As proof of that, in the 1930s a Californian oil company reported that turkey vultures were unwittingly pinpointing leaking gas pipes for them. Reacting to the faint traces of ethyl mercaptan naturally occurring in petroleum gas, the turkey vultures were gathering at the sites of any leaks, irresistibly drawn to them by an aroma they associated with the carrion and dead bodies that were their normal diet.

With an ugly, bleeding, foul-smelling and partly necrotic tumour almost filling her mouth, the prognosis for Kathleen was far from good, but we could not have predicted her reaction to that, because patients can react to a diagnosis of cancer in very different ways. Some are determined to fight it and continue having treatments, chemotherapy and radiotherapy, no matter how bleak their prospects might be. Some prefer not to be told how serious their condition has become, while others absorb the information and then make the decision to refuse any further treatment, preferring to devote their remaining time and energy to settling their affairs and spending their last days with their loved ones – and, when the time comes, saying a proper farewell to them.

Because of the pain and damage to her tongue, Kathleen had

not said much on her first visit to my consulting rooms, but her granddaughter, sitting next to her and holding her hand, was giving me the message loud and clear from the very start that Kathleen and her family wanted to get the problem fixed. Kathleen herself never specifically said that to me but she did subsequently confide in her clinical nurse specialist, Andrea, a woman I hold in the highest regard for her ability to empathize with her patients, build a strong bond with them, and speak quietly and discreetly to them when necessary. Kathleen told Andrea that her biggest fear was that the cancer would eventually suffocate her. It was heading in that direction because the tumour had grown so large that she was having to sit with her mouth open and push her tongue forward to get enough air into her lungs, and this also meant that sleep was difficult for her – on the nights when she could get any sleep at all. Despite all the analgesia we gave her, the cancer was also extremely painful for her, because if you attempt to speak or swallow your tongue has to move, and given that most of her tongue had been replaced by a tumour, that was agonizing for her.

It was at once clear that the only possibility for a cure was to remove as much as possible of the tumour. Unfortunately, the imaging we had showed that the cancer had already spread to the glands in her neck, certainly on one side and possibly on the other. So we would need to treat her by removing those lymph nodes as well, and evaluate whether it had also spread outside the capsules of the lymph glands into the surrounding tissue. If that was the case she was unlikely to survive without chemotherapy and radiotherapy, and to be effective that had to happen within a few weeks of the operation. If not, the cancer would inevitably recur, with fatal consequences.

Right from the outset, what was in my mind when I was thinking about managing Kathleen's condition was whether at her age, in her weakened condition, she would be able to stand all the treatment. In any event, it was my absolute and clear conviction that the best way to control her pain and stop her from dying horrifically of bleeding from the mouth or suffocation was to remove the tumour from her tongue.

Long experience had taught me that the best reconstruction of the tongue would be with a large free tissue transfer, for example from the thigh. By excising the tumour but preserving the muscles above the voice box and the hyoid bone (the U-shaped bone above your voice box that is always fractured if someone is strangled, thus revealing the cause of death to forensic pathologists in a post-mortem), she would still be able to elevate that part of her throat and push that thick pad of transplanted tissue out of the way so that she could swallow. In fact, as long as we could preserve the constrictor muscles at the very back of her tongue and the muscle tube that makes up the throat (which looks like three flowerpots stacked inside each other: the superior, middle and inferior constrictor), her ability to swallow would not be impaired.

Even if we did achieve a complete cure of the cancer and Kathleen was strong enough to survive the aggressive treatment needed to do so, it would not only affect her quality of life in the short term, beyond that it would also have a considerable impact on her prospects. I knew that because recent research had given us a much fuller understanding of the long-term consequences of chemotherapy. Although the therapy might control the primary cancer, when researchers tracked such cases over a period of five years from the date of the operation they discovered that many patients died from other causes during that period – heart attacks and other old-age-related conditions – that had occurred in them much earlier than normal because of the premature general body damage caused by their chemotherapy. That was the price that had to be paid by the patient for controlling the cancer that way. So, looking to the future, we have to find better, less damaging forms of treatment.

Before operating on Kathleen we went through all the discussion and work-up process, including quite a terse exchange of views with the oncologists, who were concerned about the overall outcome of the surgery and the subsequent treatment. I could understand their reluctance to accept it as the right course of treatment for her, because their role would only begin after we had got Kathleen safely through her operation. At that point we would pass her on to them and, without saying it, the expectation was that they should 'fix her up'. That might well have proved an impossible task in her case because of her general frailty and the impact of the surgery on her overall state of health – and if anyone dies within thirty days of completing a course of chemotherapy it is seen as a big black mark against the oncologists. The immediate conclusion in cases like that is that they ought to have judged their patient's condition better and not subjected a dying person to the additional trauma and side-effects of chemo, which would not have saved their life and might quite possibly have hastened their demise. Nonetheless my judgement, backed by the rest of my team, was that in Kathleen's particular circumstances surgery was the best and indeed the only option, even if it ultimately became a 'good death' procedure.

Before the operation took place I had a very careful

conversation with Kathleen, just the two of us alone together. I perched on the chair next to her bed and placed my hand on the back of hers, just so that there was some direct human contact between us. I wanted to make sure that she did not have any residual concerns that she had not felt able to voice in front of her family. I also had to be absolutely certain that she was making a fully informed decision about the best way to move forward. In such circumstances I had to act not just as her surgeon, proposing what I felt would be the best course of treatment for her, but also as devil's advocate too, pointing out all the potential pitfalls and the worst-case scenarios.

'We're in a very difficult situation, Kathleen,' I told her. 'My worry is that this tumour might bleed, but it's also proving to be very difficult to get your pain under control and the best way for us to do that is to take away that big lump on your tongue. But the worry then is that the operation may have complications and side-effects, and I'm sorry to bring it up, but we both have to consider together the possibility that a lady like you, at your age and in these circumstances, may not survive the process.'

There was no hesitation at all before she replied, 'I understand that, doctor. I trust you completely and I want you to take the lump away.'

So she was explicit about that, and if I needed any more reassurance Andrea provided it after her own further conversation with Kathleen. As a clinical nurse specialist Andrea was under a completely different chain of command at the hospital and, although integral to the cancer team, was not part of the surgical team that would be performing the operation. Nor was she someone who would agree to a particular course of treatment just to please the consultant who was proposing it. That was important, because it is often said that some staff, just like some patients – and that particularly applies to the recruitment of patients for clinical trials – will just go along with something because they want to please their doctors and not annoy or upset them, without necessarily understanding what they're signing up to. However, from Andrea's private discussions with her it was absolutely clear that Kathleen's main fear was that she would die horribly from suffocation, and whatever the consequences might be, she wanted the operation to ensure that did not happen.

That reassurance direct from Kathleen herself, backed up by Andrea, took away any residual anxiety I might have been feeling about the course of action we were about to embark on. The patient, her family and the members of the surgical team were all pulling in the same direction; we all shared the belief that this was the right thing to do. There were still one or two people with reservations, though not in the medical team, who either kept their thoughts to themselves or just discussed them quietly, because they fully understood the issue: either we carried out the procedure or Kathleen would die in agony. Those voicing doubts were some of the nursing team who, not having fully processed the information about Kathleen's condition and her own fears and wishes, felt that we shouldn't be operating on her at all.

When the day of the operation dawned, the procedure went very well. The first stage was what we call a 'visor drop down' procedure. To ensure that the resulting scar was in the least visible place, we made a continuous incision from behind the ear, following the jawline under the chin, and up behind the other ear, effectively marking out three sides of a rounded-off square.

We then peeled back the neck and facial tissue, lifting the skin and the underlying fascia out of the way. After removing lymph glands from the top of both sides of Kathleen's neck, we were able to access the tumour on her tongue, knowing that when we had resected that and transplanted a flap of tissue from else-where on her body to replace the missing part of her tongue, we could simply drop the 'visor' of facial skin back down, reattach it and, once the scars had healed, her face would be returned to its previous appearance.

We had to be careful how we dealt with the digastric muscle, which enables us to elevate our throats and swallow, because of the way it attaches to the bone of the lower jaw. If I had just removed that muscle from Kathleen's jawbone it would have been very difficult to reattach it, so instead I cut out a piece of bone from the inside of the lower jaw, at the front, under the tongue, still with the muscle attached to it, which made it much easier to reattach afterwards. When we had completed the exci-sion of the tumour, we simply had to drill a hole through the piece of bone and a slightly larger hole through the jaw and then use a 'lag-screw' to pull the two pieces together, leaving the muscle once more securely attached.

We resected the cancer with a good margin to remove any spread of microscopic cancer cells, but leaving sufficient muscle at the back of Kathleen's tongue to allow for normal speech and swallowing functions, because fortunately the tumour had not gone too far back. But worryingly, as soon as we began resecting the tumour, we could at once see the extra spread of cancer beyond it. The next step was to take away the remaining lymph glands from the neck, and this part did not hold good news either. A lot of tissue surrounding the glands was hard and stuck down, suggesting that cancer was already present in them as well and, as we had feared, had already spread outside the capsules of the lymph glands. To say the least, that was not a good sign.

Kathleen would need to have chemotherapy and radiotherapy to eradicate any remaining traces of tumour. That had to happen within six weeks if it was going to be effective, because any longer than this and the benefit of these treatments is lost and the cancer will recur. So our post-operative task was to get her well enough for radiotherapy to happen. However, I had made sure that all the members of our surgical, medical and nursing teams were left in no doubt at all about our objectives and my belief – and it was one shared by the surgical and medical teams – that even if Kathleen's eventual recovery proved to be too slow for chemotherapy and radiotherapy to be possible, it was still the right course of action. If all we had achieved was to improve the end of her life and allow her to die in dignity and without unnecessary discomfort, that would still be a very worthwhile outcome.

The tumour void was filled with a lateral thigh flap taken from about halfway between the kneecap and the front of the hip bone, with one of the descending deep blood vessels from the thigh. We reconstructed her tongue, microsurgically re-attached the tiny blood vessels supplying and draining it to those we had prepared in her neck, and saw that it was flowing beautifully. We put on the microprobe monitors, closed her up, and exchanged high-fives at the end of a very successful procedure. The cancer had been removed and Kathleen was looking great, with all her advance monitoring parameters satisfactory.

Kathleen had a tracheostomy (surgical airway) as part of her operation so she couldn't speak for the first few days after leaving theatre. When we removed the plastic tube from the hole in her neck and covered it, she could speak again. Even though we'd removed most of her native tongue and replaced it with a bulky flap from her thigh, she sounded just like herself, albeit with a slight lisp, as though the front of her tongue was stuck down. I had told Kathleen in my best Billy Connolly-style delivery before the operation, 'And if I put in some careful extra stitches at the back you'll get a Scottish accent too!' It brought a burst of laughter from her.

Like any other post-operative patient, Kathleen's recovery did not solely depend on the efficacy of the surgery, it also required meticulous attention to detail by the nursing team on the ward. Their care was excellent, but though the early post-operative signs for Kathleen were good, problems started to arise almost at once, beginning in the week following surgery. As well as her cancer, she also had scleroderma, a connective tissue disorder that leads to an abnormality of the cells that make fibres. It can cause tightening of the mouth and difficulty in swallowing, accompanied by fingernail damage, hands that turn into claws and calcinosis (the formation of calcium deposits) in the skin. Kathleen had whole body changes because of this auto-immune disorder and it was also affecting her lungs by making them fibrosed. The concern for us was that when a patient's lungs are slightly fibrosed it makes them more prone to damage when we are ventilating them mechanically during surgery.

When a machine pushes gas into your lungs, although the tidal volume – the amount of gas that's pushed in and out – is controlled very carefully to ensure that it replicates the natural process as closely as possible, the volume is the same as when you're breathing for yourself, but the pressures are not. As a result, under ventilation, every time the alveoli – the tiny little cauliflower-shaped sacs inside the lungs that allow the exchange of oxygen and carbon dioxide between the lungs and the bloodstream – are inflated and deflated, you get tiny amounts of inflammation in them as an adverse reaction to the pressures. Those tiny amounts of micro-lung damage do not happen when you are breathing naturally for yourself but under anaesthesia are very difficult to avoid.

Combined with the effects of her lung fibrosis, her time on the ventilator while we were operating had produced some lung damage that made it difficult for Kathleen to breathe and left her even more prone to chest infections. It eventually reached the point where she was no longer strong enough to breathe for herself, and in order to keep her alive we had to put her back on a ventilator. If she was to make a full recovery, at some point we would have to take her off the ventilator again, and the sooner that happened the better. Our hope was that a few more days' recuperation would allow her to build up enough strength to be able to breathe naturally on her own. But there was no guarantee that would be the case.

The term for taking that ventilator support away is 'weaning', and the best chance of weaning successfully is if you have a tracheostomy tube surgically in place, because that cuts down the amount of 'dead space' you have to fill with air every time you breathe. As you take each breath in and out, about 150 millilitres of air is taken into the mouth and throat that does not actually get to the lungs at all and is merely expelled again as you breathe out. If we take that amount of air out of the equation by inserting a tracheostomy tube in the throat, by-passing the mouth and the upper part of the throat, we reduce the amount of dead space the air has to fill and therefore cut down the effort the patient needs to make in order to breathe. Kathleen had already had a tracheostomy as part of the preparation for the primary operation, so it was a straightforward matter to restore it, although it meant we had removed her voice again.

As the weeks went by, all our attempts to wean her off the ventilator ended in failure. Whenever she was taken off it, she had to go straight back on again because she was unable to breathe unaided. Still hoping that she would recover enough strength, we waited a few more days and then tried again, but once more, as soon as she was taken off the ventilator, she had to go straight back on it.

We went past the six-week cut-off point for her treatment with chemotherapy and radiotherapy to begin, and although, apart from the weakness in her lungs, she had healed well, Kathleen was still nowhere near fit enough to begin chemotherapy because she still needed continuing ventilator support and was still in Intensive Care. More weeks went by without her being able to come off the machine and eventually we reached the point where she herself realized that the situation was hopeless, and she told Andrea and the care team looking after her 'I've had enough', and asked to be taken off the ventilator.

Although she had expressed that very clearly, for clinical and ethical reasons we had to be absolutely sure that she had the mental capacity to understand the decision she was making and what the consequences of it would be. Kathleen was therefore seen by the hospital's consultant in clinical psychology who, among other conditions, dealt with patients with Alzheimer's and other forms of dementia. Having assessed Kathleen, the clinical neuro-psychologist concluded that she was not in any way lacking the mental capacity to make an informed decision about her own care.

When I went to see her, she also expressed herself quite clearly to me, saying, 'I just don't want this machine any more.'

'That means you won't be able to breathe, Kathleen. Do you understand that?'

'Yes.'

'What do you want to do?'

'I want to go home.'

The problem was that she could not get home without the ventilator, but we could not send it with her, and that meant that she would probably not even survive to reach her home. We had a final discussion one lunchtime, with Kathleen, me and my registrar, the Intensive Care consultant and his registrar, Andrea and members of Kathleen's close family all present. I found it terribly difficult because, while dealing with death and dying has always been part of doctors' and surgeons' work, it is not often that a surgeon – and especially a cancer surgeon – will be present at, or very close to, the actual moment of death. Even if things haven't gone well with a cancer treatment, sudden death is unusual, and if the patient subsequently dies, it's more likely to be a controlled, cared-for death in a palliative care setting, or ideally at their home.

In such cases, although I wouldn't actually be present, I would be aware of the sequence of events, and of course saddened by them. For me, a nagging feeling of professional failure always accompanies a death, and a period of critical reflection. Did we do everything right? Did we do everything we could have done, or do anything that we shouldn't have done?

The day we had the discussion with Kathleen, I had my usual overbooked hurly-burly of a morning clinic with lots of things going on – 'Why is this person here? Have I seen him before? Who referred him? Who accepted the referral?' The normal bedlam, in other words. And in the midst of all that, Andrea came in and said in her soft South Wales accent, 'You haven't forgotten that we're going down to the ward to see Kathleen at lunchtime, have you?'

I was concerned that there might have been some issue with her care or treatment that either I'd not been informed about or had simply forgotten, but she told me that we were really just going down to say goodbye.

So we went down to the ward, where we found Kathleen surrounded by her family, including her two sons and her grand-children. I had my last conversation with her – and there is no clearer moment to contemplate death and the hereafter than when faced with a patient who is about to pass away. Although full of people and machines, the room was suddenly very quiet. I took in everything: the grey-painted walls and high ceiling, the smell of antiseptic in my nose (different from that in the ICU), the beeping and gentle whooshing sounds on my right, and Kathleen's family on my left. Kathleen herself was right in front of me, and looking intently at me. She seemed very slight, a wee lady floating in a sea of crisp white bed linen, with her hands resting on top of the sheets.

Once more I had to question her, just to make absolutely sure that she still understood the ramifications of her decision, had not had a last-minute change of mind, and knew beyond all doubt that if we took her off the ventilator she would struggle to breathe on her own.

She couldn't speak because of the tracheostomy but she nodded or wrote her answers on a small whiteboard. She wrote that she understood, and still wanted to go home.

'Our worry is that you won't survive if we do that, Kathleen.'

'I know,' she wrote. 'That's all right.'

I looked to her family for confirmation, and though there were tears and sadness, of course, they made it clear that they would abide by her wish.

Kathleen had always been quite cheeky with me, often rolling her eyes at some of the things her family or her care team said, and astonishingly she was still doing that, even at this sombre moment. I took both of her hands in mine and said, 'OK then, Kathleen. I think it's a very reasonable decision for you to have made, though it's very likely that is what is going to happen, but one way or the other, we're definitely going to get you home, although it may be that you will have passed away before that happens. You understand that?'

'I understand,' she wrote.

I have not often found myself holding the hands of someone who is going to die in a few minutes and I found it very difficult to control my emotions. But I had to be the strong, certain character who could give her and her family a little confidence. While I was talking to her, I had to pause a few times to stop my voice from cracking. The last words I said to her were 'OK then, I'll see you soon.'

I had worried about how Kathleen's family might react to her choice and her imminent death as a result of it, but they were a lovely bunch of people, a loving, caring family who just wanted the best for her. Whatever their personal grief, if she had decided that she had had enough and wanted to go, they accepted that and supported her right to choose the time and manner of her passing.

From my experience, the most difficult times we have in such situations is often with those who have not seen their dying relative for years. They turn up at the bedside and, perhaps through feelings of guilt at not having made more effort to see them when they were alive, launch into diatribes against the medical and surgical staff for our failure to save their relative's life. In this case, there was none of that. We shared the sadness of Kathleen's family, but we knew that it was what she wanted and that we had done everything we could, first to try to save her life, and then, when that had not proved possible, to make her passing as peaceful and pain-free as it could be.

The staff turned off Kathleen's ventilator soon after I left her bedside and sadly, as we had feared, she did not survive to reach her home. She passed away peacefully, still in the hospital, that afternoon with her family around her. A good death. I got the message that she had died from Andrea in the middle of my hectic afternoon clinic and I stopped what I was doing for a few moments to reflect.

Later I spoke with the senior trainees, recapping decisions made and treatment given. I said to them, 'Do you ever wonder what there is after this? Kathleen knows now.' We talked a little more, touching on Epicurean philosophy ('I was not, I am, I will not be, I will not worry') and on other beliefs: my Catholic upbringing with its tradition of hell (which always seems like so much effort to produce), purgatory and heaven, Hindu reincarnation and Islam. The hospital we were in had 163 different languages spoken within it and multiple different religious traditions. My sadness that Kathleen's treatment had ultimately been unsuccessful was tempered by the knowledge that things had ended well for her, her death being a gentle slip from consciousness among family, not a suffocating, bleeding, painful indignity.

It had been a very difficult situation but I was certain that we had done our very best for her, and that surgery was definitely the right thing. Had Kathleen got to the stage of having chemo-therapy and radiotherapy she might not have survived it anyway, and would certainly have been made very sick by it. As it was, hers was a calm and dignified end. Kathleen's relatives kept her wish and took her home after her death, where she lay in state overnight, watched over by family members. She was a lovely lady but she was tired and had had enough and decided it was time to go.

Morbidity and Mortality meetings, or 'the meetings about sur-gical events with negative outcomes' as I'm sometimes tempted to rename them, are held by all hospitals. They are supposed to be an opportunity to discuss what went right and what went wrong in the cases we have treated, so that we can learn lessons from them and the care we offer can be improved in the future. That is how they operate at most hospitals, but unfortunately at one or two others these meetings are more like rotten-fruit-throwing contests. That is mostly down to the clash between the contrasting attitudes of consultants and senior doctors that might be characterized as a split between those whose motto is cui bono – literally 'for whose benefit' – and those who are much more likely to have 'follow the money' on their coat of arms, working in institutions where private practice is prevalent.

In less supportive institutions, someone whose patient has

suffered complications can find themselves being challenged, criticized and ridiculed by their peers, whereas the Morbidity and Mortality meeting really ought to be an exercise where we all go through the process together and think in a considered and supportive fashion. Could this have been avoided? Did anything not happen that should have? What might we do differently next time? And so on.

The day when Kathleen's case was due to be reviewed happened to be a day when I was out of the country at a head and neck surgery conference. My consultant colleague, Abdul, couldn't be there either, so a registrar had to present Kathleen's case for me. I had some concerns about that, worrying that the audience there might be less than supportive of a trainee who had been asked to stand in for a consultant, particularly as, faced with a room full of specialists and consultants in other disciplines, she did not have the experience, seniority or security of status to rebut any criticisms they might make. I felt that the situation could have been unfair for her, so I took the time to brief her very carefully beforehand. I gave her the clinical photographs of the massive tumour in Kathleen's mouth and photographs of Kathleen herself, showing how old and frail she was, and said, 'Whatever you do, be certain to show them these pictures. In fact, make sure you start with them.'

As it turned out, unlike some high-level institutions where I've worked where there was a great deal of competition and ego, my fears for my registrar were groundless on this occasion, because as soon as she stopped speaking, the unanimous verdict of the assembled consultants was 'Well, we'd have had the operation as well. Next case.'

11

CASES SUCH AS Kathleen's highlight the ethical dilemmas doctors and surgeons often face, above and beyond the purely clinical considerations of how to deal with a patient. The Hippocratic Oath laid out the basic ethical principles of the practice of medicine almost 2,500 years ago, and several modern versions have been produced, but until the middle of the twentieth century moral quandaries rarely troubled doctors for long, mainly because it was assumed, almost without question, that what was clinically possible was also ethically acceptable. Patients' opinions about their treatment were rarely sought by doctors and even more rarely volunteered. This 'Doctor Knows Best' belief was so widely accepted, by doctors and patients alike, that it became a cliché, but it did not long survive the Second World War. Revulsion at the role of doctors in Nazi Germany who experimented upon and killed defenceless captives led to a strengthening of medical codes of ethics and the official oversight of the profession, and in the second half of the twentieth century and into the twenty-first, the belief in the near-infallibility of doctors' judgement has increasingly been challenged by a growing awareness of, and attention to, the rights of individuals and minorities.

The definitive endpoint of the Doctor Knows Best era may well have been the case of Murray v. McMurchy in 1949. While performing a Caesarean section upon an anaesthetized patient, the surgeon discovered a tumour. Believing that if the patient again became pregnant it would endanger her life and that enduring a second surgical procedure would also be injurious to her, the surgeon took the decision to tie the woman's Fallopian tubes, but he did so without first seeking her consent. When she discovered that he had done this, the woman sued him for negligence and won her case. While the judge found that the surgeon had made the correct clinical decision, his failure to consult his patient and take her views into account amounted to negligence.

The modern code of medical ethics, overseen by the various Royal Colleges and by the General Medical Council, encompasses what are known as the 'Four Principles'. These state that doctors should always:

1. Do good and not do harm.
2. Respect their patients' opinions and decisions about their medical condition and its treatment.
3. Respect patients' autonomy over decisions that directly affect them.
4. Respect the principle of justice in healthcare, i.e. fairness in the allocation of medical resources and of patients' access to treatment.

However, the latter principle, the foundation stone of the National Health Service in 1948, is increasingly coming under pressure from financial constraints and the ever-expanding role of the private sector within the NHS.

It is arguable that doctors in the modern era are required to adhere to higher moral standards than other professions. Not only are we expected to be technically excellent, good at our jobs, we're also expected to be morally excellent – good human beings too. Perhaps that helps to explain the shock and outrage on the rare occasions when a doctor 'goes bad'. Partly as a result of events such as the Harold Shipman case and partly owing to the end of the 'age of deference' and the rise of individual awareness and assertiveness, doctors now find themselves under ever greater scrutiny and pressure, not always with beneficial consequences.

Anecdotal evidence suggests that the practice by some doctors of cutting short some of their terminally ill patients' lives – for example, by administering a very high dose of morphine – was once relatively common. Although never legal, it might well have been seen by doctors and patients, and by the patients' families, who had often known their family doctor all their lives, as a victimless crime, a humane way of easing the suffering of a dying relative.

Whether as a result of a wider knowledge of codes of medical ethics, the tighter control and scrutiny of the prescription of powerful drugs, the fear of exposure and legal action or, to a lesser extent, the change in the way that most GPs run their practices today, making the lifelong connection between a particular family and a particular doctor far less prevalent than in the past, a doctor is much less likely to resort to such measures today. Some of those who have done so have been prosecuted and convicted.

However, under palliative care, patients in the final stages of a terminal illness such as cancer are still prescribed high doses of pain-relieving drugs, even though it is known that they will shorten the remaining span of their life, often by depressing the respiratory function. It is an example of the law of double effect, first identified by Thomas Aquinas, which states that a good action may also have a secondary bad consequence, without negating the value of the original action. Doctors would argue that accelerating their patient's death was not their prime motivation in prescribing the drugs, rather that it was an unfortunate but necessary and inevitable consequence of the primary good aim: to mitigate the patient's pain.

The complexity of the moral judgements doctors must make has only continued to increase. Ethical questions are rarely straightforward and require a careful balancing of clinical imperatives with the patient's wishes, but these considerations are doubly difficult when a patient's judgement may be qualified or impaired by disease, illness, disability, or by their youth or age. Even more complicated are cases where, because of mental illness, a debilitating condition or extreme physical pain, a patient's ability to make informed decisions may fluctuate over time, even from day to day.

Doctors have to make life-changing decisions all the time, but their patients sometimes have to do so too. Patients, not doctors, must decide whether they wish to terminate a pregnancy, whether to decline treatment on religious grounds, whether to refuse further treatment for a terminal illness, or whether to actively promote their own death by asking for the ventilator or dialysis machine that is keeping them alive to be switched off – a decision that in other circumstances would be described as suicide. In all those cases, the patients' wishes must be paramount, but only, as in Kathleen's case, if they are assessed to be sufficiently autonomous and mentally competent to make those decisions, having understood all the consequences of them.

The giant strides that have been made in terms of technique in every branch of medicine in modern times have made such ethical dilemmas even more acute. Advances in technology mean that chronically disabled babies who without question would have died at birth in previous eras can now be saved. The average person's lifespan has also been greatly extended. But in all these cases the question of 'quality of life' assumes ever greater importance. To put it crudely: just because we have the skills and knowledge to carry out a particular procedure does not mean that we should. This places a burden on the medical profession now that used never to be there.

The ethical issues that are involved in these cases are often terrifyingly complex. For example, who would wish to have the onerous responsibility of having to decide whether or not to devote huge amounts of hospital time and scarce resources to keeping alive a premature disabled baby who, if he or she survives at all, will be in constant pain throughout their life as a result of those disabilities? At the other end of life, who would want to have to decide whether or not to keep resuscitating an elderly and extremely ill patient suffering recurring bouts of pneumonia, and who may even have expressed a wish to die?

The wishes of patients, where they are able to express them, are vital of course, but so too may be those of their close relatives. And the questions we doctors must resolve are often agonizing. If a procedure will extend a patient's lifespan but do nothing to alleviate their suffering, should it be carried out? Decisions in such cases must always be collective, with the doctor (or more often today a multi-disciplinary team of doctors and specialist nurses) advising on the best clinical course of action and the consequences if it is followed – and if it is not – but with a fully informed and autonomous patient having the right to accept the treatment or reject it in the light of their own wishes and personal circumstances.

Not all of the ethical dilemmas I have faced were the result of having to deal with purely medical problems. One patient, Faith, was a Jehovah's Witness who, as a result of a tumour in her upper jaw, needed an orbital exenteration – the surgical removal of the eyeball and surrounding tissues, including the eyelids, muscles, nerves and fatty tissue around the eye, together with the cancer in her upper jaw and air sinus. However, her religious beliefs led her to refuse to countenance the transfusions that would normally be regarded as essential to counter the blood loss she would suffer during such an operation. This was especially true if we were to reconstruct using her hip bone and abdominal muscles – those patients always need blood from others. After trying and failing to persuade her to change her mind, I reluctantly acceded to her wishes, and after much thought and discussion with members of my team and with consultants in my own and other specialities, I found a way to operate with only minimal bleeding, by reconstructing her face without using a flap from her hip and tummy. I explained to Faith that she would need an obturator – an extended type of upper denture carrying teeth – to block the hole in the middle of her face up to her now empty eye socket. She told me this was entirely fine 'as long as I can still say Jehovah', but the constraints would make it an unusually stressful procedure – for me as well as the patient.

When I went to see her on the ward before going into theatre Faith greeted me with a smile. I explained again how worried I was about the operation if she would not accept blood and my fear that she might not survive. 'Professor McCaul,' she said, 'I'm so confident and so delighted because, you see, God has sent you to me.'

'That's true,' I said, 'but on the other hand, he has also sent you to me. The Lord giveth with one hand and he taketh away with the other . . .'

She did a double-take and then burst out laughing.

Before going ahead with the operation we obtained the loan of a 'cell-saver' from the Brompton Hospital. This is a piece of equipment that is normally used in thoracic surgery, where there is a lot of blood loss. If the patient is bleeding, you can use the device to suction up the blood and put it through the machine, which cleans it up so you can put it back into the patient. It's difficult to use during head and neck surgery, and in any case it's always been hard to convince people involved in cancer surgery to use it because of the fear that, along with their blood, you might be reintroducing cancer cells to the patient's body. But the fact is that cancer patients have cancer cells in their circulation anyway and those cells don't actually do anything harmful unless the tumour progresses, or, in Darwinian fashion, the cells evolve the right sort of sticky stuff on their surfaces – the cell surface receptors – to begin the formation of another tumour mass elsewhere in the body. In any case, the filters on the cell-saver device mostly eliminate cancer cells.

So, following Faith's decision – principled or obstinate, depending on your point of view – we obtained the cell-saver machine together with the specialist technician who accompanied it, like the ones who work the by-pass machines for cardiac surgery. However, it was only worth using the machine if there was going to be more than 350 millilitres of blood to recycle, and thanks to our meticulous care – and, it has to be said, a generous dose of good fortune – the whole of the resection of her neck, mid-face and eye, which you would normally expect to bleed a lot, saw her lose less than 350 millilitres. So the

technician and her machine had a wasted journey, at least from
the point of view of actually recycling Faith's blood, but I certainly felt safer with the reassurance of this safety net for her,
and I could feel the relief from the surgical and nursing team
too. To restrict blood loss to such a low level was almost miraculous . . . so just what a deeply religious person like Faith would
have expected!

In my post-operative reflection, I did have to wonder if we
could achieve similar reductions in blood loss by operating
with such extreme care the rest of the time, or whether Faith's
case really had benefited from great good fortune – or, in her
view, divine intervention.

Providing the patient is in a reasonable state of general health,
the majority of my cases have positive outcomes, even if, like
Kathleen's, an operation does no more than ensure that they
have an end of life that is free from fear and pain. But there are
some ultra-aggressive forms of cancer that can prove impossible to treat. Philip was one such case, a man in his late fifties
who had recently retired from the police force. He was a very
modest and self-effacing chap who had originally gone to his
GP complaining of a headache and pain in the middle third of
his face. He saw his doctor about it on several subsequent occasions over a period of about four months.

He was suffering from sinusitis which did not respond to
four or five courses of antibiotics, and really, when it didn't
respond to the second set he should have been referred for further investigation straight away. If two courses of antibiotics
have not solved a problem, another two or three are not going
to do so either, and if there is a cancer hiding in the mid-face

inside the air sinus you are not going to find it without a scan. Since a CT scan takes thirty seconds and is really cheap, even if the NHS is strapped for cash – and it always is – there is no excuse for not doing a precautionary scan.

However, he had not been referred to me until well after the point when he should have been, and tragically had only been diagnosed at a very late stage when a tumour had already started to come down through the roof of his mouth and his nose, causing blood to seep from it. By then he was experiencing a great deal of discomfort, and although the X-ray imaging didn't show it, I thought it very likely that the tumour was already heading towards his skull base. If it reached there and went through, it would almost inevitably have fatal consequences.

Philip and his wife were sitting in dignified silence when I went into the consulting room, but I soon detected a quiet but powerful sense of desperation coming from them, especially Philip's wife, which created a pressure on my chest. I wanted to fix this for him. At first as we sat there, prior to discussing his symptoms in detail and the possible courses of treatment available to him, I was trying to put him at ease a little by making some more general conversation, but he was quite reticent and didn't say very much at all. He told me that his wife was a nurse (always an important fact to be aware of) so we talked about our experiences with the NHS for a while and then, still trying to draw him out a little, I asked, 'So what rank did you get to in the police then?', expecting that over maybe four decades his career would have progressed.

'Police Constable,' he said firmly.

'Oh, right,' I said, but I can't entirely have managed to keep the surprise from my voice because he just looked at me in silence for a moment before adding, 'I just took a great deal of pleasure from doing the job and seeing it done as well as possible. That's what I enjoyed: doing my job fairly and doing it well.'

I felt a bit abashed by that. I'd assumed he'd have been ambitious to climb the career ladder, as most people are, but it turned out that he had never been motivated by money or rank at all. All he had ever wanted to do was serve the community as an ordinary police constable, doing the job to the absolute best of his ability. That kind of dedication and self-effacement is something you do not hear enough about nowadays, even though in the medical field there are many nurses and nursing auxiliaries who are equally dedicated to serving their communities. It was inspiring to hear him talk about his work that way. He had devoted his entire working life to his community, and now I felt it was up to us, as part of that community, to do something for him.

Having talked to him a while longer and found out all I could about his symptoms and the cause of them, the first priority was to get his pain under control because, although Philip was a very stoic man, he was suffering terribly. Fortunately there is a well-established pain control ladder, approved by the World Health Organization. Under that WHO guidance, painkilling drugs are to be taken orally where possible, and are most effective when given at regular intervals of three to six hours 'by the clock', rather than on demand. Where necessary, to help calm the patient's fear and anxiety, the analgesia (pain relief) can also be accompanied by 'adjuvant drugs' that are used to treat a side-effect or manage a co-existing symptom.

The first step on the pain control ladder, simple analgesia, is paracetamol. Everybody knows about paracetamol – there's probably some in every bathroom cupboard in the land – nonetheless it is a drug that is underrated by the general public. It works on the spinal cord and the brain, specifically the peri-aqueductial grey matter (the brain's control centre for pain modulation) and the substantia gelatinosa (the interface between the forebrain and the lower brain stem), which plays a major role in the body's response to internal stresses such as pain and external stresses such as the threat of violence – the 'fight or flight' response, in other words. So paracetamol is a very effective pain relief agent. People often say 'Oh, it never works for me, it never touches my pain', but all that means is that the dose wasn't high enough. And of equal importance is the fact that, if you have paracetamol as the baseline, it greatly reduces the amount of other very strong, high-side-effect medications that we have to use.

The next tier, but always building on the foundation provided by paracetamol, is the adjuvant group of drugs, like ibuprofen and diclofenac (these are non-steroidal anti-inflammatory drugs, known as NSAIDS for short) and other nerve-modifying agents such as gabapentin and pregabalin, which alter how nerves transmit pain signals.

The next level above the adjuvant group is the start of the opioids (the proper word for morphine-related drugs, not opiates, which refers to the receptors in the body). Codeine is one of the weaker opioids and tramadol is a medium-strength one, but even that is still only 20 per cent of the strength of morphine and diamorphine.

If we need stronger opioids as the next rung on the pain relief ladder, we increasingly use newer, synthetic ones such as fentanyl or oxycodone, rather than morphine or diamorphine. Fentanyl is used a lot in anaesthesia because it has a rapid onset and is very effective indeed. It's fifty to a hundred times more potent than morphine but has a very short half-life; in other words, it passes through the system very quickly, being rapidly metabolized in the liver and excreted in the patient's urine. So there is much less of the hangover effect and the nausea you get with other drugs, and it's much safer for certain patients, particularly those who have renal (kidney) impairment.

The reason for that is that drugs are modified and detoxified in your liver and then passed out through your urine in a process known as glucuronidation, but if the kidneys aren't working very well, some of the metabolites of morphine, for example, instead of being disposed of in the urine, get released back into the body's circulation, and they still work. So those drugs can catch you out, and if someone has renal impairment, it can lead to potentially fatal levels of toxicity. That is why the newer drugs like fentanyl are safer than the morphine and diamorphine we would traditionally have used because they are excreted so much faster. Fentanyl has been in the news because abuse of it by drug addicts, often in combination with heroin, has led to a number of deaths, but used in a controlled medical environment it is perfectly safe and, as I said, very effective.

So managing Philip's pain was the first priority, but using the pain control ladder, that was something we could fix almost overnight. I prescribed what I thought would be the right amount of analgesia and then sent him home for the weekend. As it was a Friday, I said to him, 'Here are the details for the on-call team, in case your pain isn't easing down the way we want it to. You can ring the number at any time, day or night, over the weekend, and if you're not feeling a lot more comfortable by Monday at the very latest we need to hear from you, so we can change your analgesia and get your pain under control.'

When we saw him again on the Monday morning there was an almost palpable air of relief about him and his wife; their confidence in our team was now growing. He was more vocal and he reported that, for the first time in weeks, he'd had a much more comfortable couple of days. Having established a satisfactory pain control regime for him, we began a series of investigations and started formulating the treatment plan he needed, which would include the removal and replacement of a large chunk of his mid-face. The first step would involve dividing the face down the middle. We would then peel back the facial tissues, exposing the underlying bone structure but preserving the skin over the surface. Then the whole mid-part of his face surrounding the tumour would have to come out and we would then be able to reconstruct the defect using a free flap from his hip. It was always a challenging procedure because of the distance between the site of the reconstruction and the artery and vein in the neck that we would use to supply and drain blood to and from the flap.

When we came to do the operation, it went very smoothly at first. We sculpted the flap perfectly to fill the void left by the excision of the tumour, the artery to it ran beautifully, and the technical aspects of the anastomosis (the sewing together) of the vein to drain it were also spot on. Sewing the two ends of the vein together is always challenging, even when looking at it down the microscope with the benefit of ten to forty times magnification, but it is something that microsurgeons do all the time, and it works well 95 per cent of the time, and more than that in my team's hands in our unit. Unfortunately, Philip's case turned out to be one of the less than 5 per cent of cases. The vein just wouldn't go, or rather it did run at first but was then blocked with a blood clot, and though we carefully clamped, opened and cleared it under the microscope, the vein kept clotting.

In the end we just couldn't get that flap to run, so we had to pull out from that and instead took some bone from the radius in his arm – the bigger bone on the outside of the arm when you're holding it palm upwards – together with the soft tissue, skin and fascia (the fatty tissue under the skin). That flap has a longer pedicle – the length of 'tubing' to connect to the neck. We transferred that to the mid-part of his face and once more the anastomosis went perfectly and the artery was flowing fine but the vein to drain the flap still kept clotting. We had five, six, maybe even seven goes at it, and at the last-ditch attempt, by which time it was seven in the morning and the sun had long since come up, the flap finally ran and, almost unbelievably, Philip at last had a functioning reconstruction. Even after all that time I still felt sharp and focused and my microsurgery was flowing, perhaps because we had already been doing it all afternoon, evening and night, though that may have been slightly illusory – a return to the sleep-deprived psychopathy I had experienced as a younger doctor.

By that time we had been operating on Philip continuously for twenty-one hours. Looking back at the procedure after-wards, you tend to think, 'Is it me? Am I really bad at this today? Was there something wrong with our set-up?' My colleague Dave Sutton, an excellent microsurgeon, and I had been working solidly together on Philip, as we had done together on many dozens of patients. Two very experienced microsurgeons, with a long and successful track record, frequently swapping roles from primary operator to assistant in order to stay fresh, performing what looked like perfect anastomosis (joins) in the blood vessels, and yet on this occasion it just would not work. We had breaks where we sat in disbelief, working through possible reasons and new strategies before scrubbing back in. At times it almost felt like a nightmare where I was scrambling up an ever steeper cliff, but slipping back and being thrown off. At one point one of our senior trainees, sensitive to this growing desperation, said, 'I hope this helps: we all know that if you two can't get it to work, no one can.' There are some syndromes that cause excessive blood clotting but to our knowledge Philip had none of them. Sometimes cancer can cause this. In the final analysis, we came to understand that the cause of the problem was not incompetence on our part but a very aggressive cancer that was causing hypercalcaemia (high blood calcium) – and in head and neck cancer that is always a bad sign – and was also pro-coagulant, causing the flap to clot.

Although that length of time under anaesthesia was far from ideal, Philip had been in good general health beforehand and had kept himself fit since retiring from the police, so his physiology could take it. We closed him up, and at that stage all looked to be going well. However, instead of the rapid recovery we were hoping for, Philip improved only very slowly after the operation.

It must have been agonizing for his wife, who as a nurse had a lot of insight into the peri-operative phase and so knew what he would be going through. She understood his suffering and his caring needs, and she was also familiar with the pain relief and the agents he was on, and knew exactly what they meant. We could all see that he just wasn't getting better in the way we would have expected, and his calcium levels kept going up. That didn't necessarily mean that his bone was being dissolved by the cancer but something was causing his hypercalcaemia, and long experience told me it was a sure sign that the cancer was a highly aggressive one and things were going to go badly for Philip.

As if in confirmation of that, he then developed a new head-ache that was very difficult to treat. I was confident that it wasn't a symptom of a tumour actually growing in his brain, because a brain tumour causes three things: pain, seizures and focal neurology – impairments of brain, spinal cord or brain func-tion. In other words, the bit of brain affected by a tumour will produce specific ramifications. So if it's in the occipital lobe at the right-hand side at the back, you get specific patches of your visual fields missing – you don't just lose the sight of the eye, you lose a particular field of vision from that eye. If the tumour is affecting the motor cortex, then a certain part of your body will be paralysed in a pattern that would make a surgeon think, 'That's brain, not nerve, nerve root, or spinal cord.'

Philip didn't have any of those problems, so it was very unlikely that we were dealing with a tumour in the brain. How-ever, that left us no wiser about what might actually be causing his hypercalcaemia and headache. So, twelve days after the ini-tial surgery, not really sure if we would find anything new, we did a fresh CT scan of his head carried out by Elizabeth Loney, who is a terrific head and neck radiologist. As soon as she had examined the results of the scan, Elizabeth told me, 'There is nothing in his brain, so that's good, but there is a tumour destroying his skull base.'

Although we had excised the tumour in his mouth and mid-face, it had already caused a cancer spread making its way back up the cranial nerves that serve the tongue, the teeth and the face, and it had begun invading and attacking his skull base, and had gone through. It was a sickening revelation because at that point I knew we had lost the battle, and I would have to give him the heart-breaking news that there was nothing further we or anyone else could do for him.

He would have been entirely justified in railing against his fate and giving full vent to his anger, cursing and swearing at me and anyone else within reach, but, remarkably, he never uttered a word of complaint. Whenever I called to see him on the ward he would be sitting up quietly in bed, but when I said 'And how are you today, Philip?' he would often say, 'Actually my headache's terrible.' Yet until that moment he would not have said a word about it to anyone.

Sadly, we could do nothing to help him except manage his pain until the inevitable end came. In fact he succumbed to the cancer very quickly. It was a typical example of a hyper-aggressive cancer that was always getting away from us, and it had taken the life of a dignified and decent man who had served the community in a dedicated and admirably self-effacing way, and who deserved much better from life than the cruel end it had in store for him.

While surgery is still the way to treat such highly aggressive cancers at the moment – even though sometimes, as in Philip's case, that surgical intervention comes too late to save a life – there are new therapies under clinical testing and development that offer some real hope for the future, like using T-cells to attack the cancer. A T-cell is a type of lymphocyte that circulates in the bloodstream and plays a key role in the immune system's response to infected or malignant cells (the 'T' stands for 'thymus', the organ in which the cells mature). In trials of the agents that produce an upregulation (increase) of immune cells, some patients with head and neck cancer are getting sick because of immune-related disorders, but these new drugs show great promise as potential treatments for them. The patients getting immune symptoms seem to be the same patients whose tumours are shrinking. Clinical trials are ongoing to assess their suitability for treatment of head and neck cancers, but early results are encouraging.

Using such drugs, we may be able to improve the body's ability to seek out and destroy cancer cells so the patient's own body could control the cancer, if we could just help to guide it – by targeting the missiles, if you like. We really have to move on with these better therapies, because for all the advances we've made we're still losing too many patients like Philip. It gives me a feeling of absolute helplessness and despair to see a CT scan like the one Elizabeth Loney made of Philip's head, and find myself thinking, 'Christ, now what?' And all too often I know that the answer, very sadly, is, 'There's nothing more we can do.'

Sometimes as I reflect on the patients I've dealt with I'll find myself thinking 'Was that too much treatment? Could we have got away with less?' because obviously the patient's best interests are served by giving him the minimum treatment necessary to cure the condition, and anything beyond that is merely increasing the risk of complications. But there are also times when an aggressive cancer is like a wildfire burning through a patient, and we will be trying one treatment after another and still will not be able to find a cure. On those occasions, my thoughts are always the reverse of those other reflections, because this time I'll be thinking 'Was that enough? Could I have done more to save him?'

12

ALTHOUGH CASES WHERE treatment was either unsuccessful or at best palliative tend to linger longest in my memory, the great majority of cases we treat end well, and the results and the long-term consequences are hugely rewarding for us and life-enhancing or even life-transforming for the patient.

One such patient, Arthur, was a forty-year-old motor mechanic, a no-nonsense Yorkshireman who ran his own small garage business. The first sign of problems for him was a small white lump in his mouth. It wasn't giving him any pain or discomfort at that stage and having shown it to his wife, Angela, he promptly forgot about it and got on with his work, but she was sufficiently concerned to phone their doctor and make an appointment for him.

When he went to see the doctor, he told Arthur, 'I don't know what that is, so we need you to see a specialist.'

Within a week, still feeling quite upbeat and unconcerned, he was seen by a specialist and had a biopsy. He went back to work, quite relaxed, and returned a week later for the results. 'It was only at that point,' he said, 'when I walked into the room and saw there were a lot of medical people waiting for me, that I thought, "We're on a tight budget here with the NHS – why are all these people here?" Only then did I realize it was much more serious than I'd thought.'

I was one of those medical people, and I explained to him

that the biopsy showed he had a tumour in his mouth and we would need to carry out further tests, CT scans and MRI scans to reassure ourselves that there was no cancer spread beyond it.

'When you told me that it was a tumour,' Arthur said, 'it didn't mean much to me at that point. It still wasn't hurting me at all and I still saw myself as a relatively young man who just cracked on with things. I didn't realize how frightening it could be.'

By the time he came to see me, just before the operation to remove the tumour, I could see that he was now well aware of what it might mean for him. I sat alongside him, rather than facing him across the desk, which I hoped would help to create the feeling in him that we were partners in this, rather than a surgeon laying down the law to his patient. He was clearly very worried about the outcome of his treatment – and as with all surgical procedures, there was obviously an element of risk attached to it – but I laid my hand on his arm and told him, 'I can't guarantee you that this will turn out well, Arthur, though obviously I hope and expect that it will, but what I can promise you is that I'll be with you every step of the way.'

Six weeks after he had first seen our team, he came in at three o'clock one Sunday afternoon, ready for surgery first thing the following morning. 'I just didn't want to go,' he later told me. 'I'd been with Angela since I was sixteen and I was now forty-one, and I was just really scared about what might happen. I'd been to see my mum that day as well – and we'd just lost my dad to cancer earlier that year, so emotions were running fairly high there.'

Nonetheless, Angela dropped him off at the hospital and then went home to look after their two sons, but promised she'd be back at seven in the morning before he went down to the operating theatre. She was there, as she'd promised, on the dot of seven. Arthur had had the pre-med, 'but that didn't really relax me,' he said, 'because by now I was just such a wreck, and I didn't want to leave Angela at all. She came with me when I was taken down to the theatre and I can remember her telling me to lie down and relax, but I couldn't stop telling her I loved her. I was still telling her that when the anaesthetic knocked me out!'

Angela burst into tears as she looked at him, asleep on the table, so I walked out of the theatre suite with her, trying to impart a few words of reassurance and promising her that we would look after him.

The operation went very well, and when Arthur came round in Intensive Care Angela was once more at his bedside. He couldn't speak because of the tracheostomy in his throat, but his smile spoke volumes. However, although everything was going well at first, and he was safely transferred from the Intensive Care Unit to the High Dependency Unit, Arthur then started to feel that there was something wrong with the tracheostomy in his throat. 'It felt really restricted,' he later told me, 'and I just couldn't breathe. I managed to get the attention of the nurse but I couldn't speak, so I couldn't tell her what was wrong and I just had to point at my throat. I can remember my heart was going at about a hundred beats a minute too, so it was just an awful experience.'

The HDU team managed to calm him and regulate his breathing, but though physically he was slowly recovering, psychologically he felt that he was getting worse. 'The following couple of days, things just went downhill,' he said. 'I'm a level-headed guy, I'm a working-class lad, I know how things are, but

I really thought I was dying. The worse I felt – and I don't know how much was in my mind and how much was the after-effects of the surgery – the worse I got. I was convinced I was dying, and I thought that all the people around me who loved me and were caring for me knew that as well, but weren't saying so.

'I was that out of it that at one point when I was asleep my mind obviously wasn't, because I felt I was floating down this black tunnel, and right at the far end there was a bright white light, like a single LED light. I'd just reached it when all of a sudden the lights came back on – I guess I'd opened my eyes at that point – and I was in the HDU in the middle of the night and it was as quiet as the grave, and I remember thinking, "Is this it? Have I died?"'

Arthur then tried to get out of bed and was pulling all the lines out, so all the monitoring machines were going crazy. The staff restrained him and called me in, and Arthur has a clear memory of me 'multi-tasking – taking your jacket off, trying to check the readings on the machines, and talking to the nursing staff while trying to calm me down as well, all at the same time!'

That proved to be his lowest point, and from then on he made excellent progress, greatly helped by his wife. 'Angela was really strong right through it,' Arthur said. 'She told me "This job's got to be done", and when I told her after the operation that I was feeling low she was having none of it. She said to me, "Arthur, this is the best day of your life. Today that cancer has gone. This is it. You're at the start, not the finish." She was right, of course, and when I got the tracheostomy out that was a massive day for me. I was still very sore but I knew then that everything that had gone on – the anaesthetic, the surgery, the drugs, the mental state I'd been in – all that was now behind me.'

When I saw him just after taking the tracheostomy out for him I said 'Morning Arthur!' and then held back, smiling broadly at him but not saying anything else.

He hesitated, nervously cleared his throat a couple of times, and then tried a response. 'Morning.' His voice was understandably croaky – not only was his throat sore from the tracheostomy, but they were the first words he'd spoken in days – but when he heard himself speak a huge smile lit up his face.

'I told you you'd get your voice back, didn't I?'

'I know you did,' he said, and tears welled up in his eyes. 'But I just thought I was going to die.'

Arthur returned for regular check-ups at first, all of which were clear, and he has now passed the five-year mark without any fresh alarms and is embracing life with a renewed appetite for everything it has to offer. 'I'm flying,' he told me. He still comes in for a check-up once a year but only because he wants to, for reassurance, not because we think it's medically necessary. He's taken up fell-running and cycling, and has done the Coast-to-Coast in one day, the Tour of Flanders and a host of other challenges to raise money for our research.

Arthur and patients like him are a heart-warming reminder that while, like all surgeons, I have a cemetery of regrets for those patients I've been unable to save, they are far outnumbered by those I and my team have been able to restore to a healthy and fulfilling life.

13

WHEN IT COMES to treating trauma patients, no matter how complex their surgery may be they almost always go on to lead a full life. There are no such certainties with cancer patients, and the treatment can sometimes be almost as difficult and painful as the disease itself. Even if a cure is achieved, the effects of the procedure on the patient's health can be long-lasting and often permanent.

A patient called Tom experienced a very difficult year when he developed a non-healing and painful open wound on the right side of his face, exposing the bone underneath. The cause took a long time to diagnose but was eventually recognized as a very rare diffused large B cell lymphoma – a white blood cell tumour – located in his lower jaw. When that was finally spotted after about fifteen biopsies in as many months, he was given six cycles of chemotherapy, and came through it; but while the chemo had damaged the lymphoma cells as it was designed to do, it had also caused severe collateral damage to the bone of his lower jaw.

Tom then had consolidation radiotherapy. It was slightly less intense than you would normally give for curative treatment of mouth or throat cancer, but because the target tissue was not in the tongue, the floor of the mouth or the throat, but the lower jaw itself, the covering skin got more of a radiation dose than usually occurs, causing severe damage to the bone and skin, including osteonecrosis – the death of the cells of the bone.

Although his cancer had been eradicated, Tom was now in terrible discomfort because the weakness of the bone had become so critical that it led to a fracture in his lower jaw. Every time the fractured bone ends moved – and it is impossible to talk, eat or swallow without moving the jaw – he was in absolutely desperate pain. As a result, he was on huge doses of morphine to deal with it.

He did some research on what was necessary to restore his jaw and face, and which surgeons might be able to do the work, then deliberately sought me out. Having explained his problem, his next words to me were 'I think you're the man for the job – are you?', to which the only reply I could give was, 'Yes, I think I am.'

Despite expressing that total confidence, I was in no doubt that it would be a very tricky condition to cure. We could not get rid of his pain by immobilizing the jaw, because such was the level of bone damage from the chemotherapy and radiotherapy that if we had tried to clamp it together with a metal plate, as we might have done in other circumstances, the bone would simply have fallen apart. The radiation he had absorbed had had the effect of prematurely ageing the cells of his jawbone, if you like, so any further trauma, even that caused by an operation to try to rectify the problem, would simply be like throwing petrol on to a smouldering fire and would only make things worse. Similarly, if we had tried to use an old-fashioned external fixator, with pins connecting a metal scaffolding surrounding his face to his jaw, the bones would simply have melted, disintegrating and falling apart at the points where the fixator was connected.

In the end we removed a large section of the damaged

jawbone and reconstructed it with a long piece of his fibula (the outer, smaller bone in the lower leg) in three sections, strengthening it with a titanium plate all the way round the jaw. We bent the titanium using a template of his own mandible that we had taken from a CT scan, so we could form an identical shape. I also took a paddle of tissue from his leg with the bone flap to form healthy tissue on the inside of his jaw and mouth.

The operation went smoothly and the flap of tissue and the transplanted bone were doing well, but Tom's problems were far from over because it soon became apparent that the remaining native tissue of his mouth to either side of the flap had been so badly damaged by chemotherapy and radiotherapy that it just wouldn't heal on to the flap. So we had a situation where the transplanted piece of his leg was mending well and looking as good as could be, but the mucosa – his tongue and the inside of his cheek – just wouldn't heal.

It was heart-breaking and agonizing for him, and it was soul-destroying for us, because no matter how perfectly we performed our surgical tasks, our patient was just not recovering in the way that we would have hoped and expected. Part of the problem was his age. This wasn't some eighteen- or twenty-year-old soldier like the ones Harold Gillies had treated, who, apart from the effects of a poor diet and too many cigarettes, were strong young physical specimens. Tom was a middle-aged man whose body had been attacked by chemotherapy and radiotherapy and as a result his tissues were in a terrible state.

Tom's case made me think of a famous statement by Ambroise Paré, a sixteenth-century French barber-surgeon who served four French kings and was not only a pioneer of surgical techniques but also of scientific method, forensic pathology and the treatment of battlefield injuries. After curing one patient's serious wound, Paré remarked, 'Je le pansai, Dieu le guérit' – 'I dressed it, God healed it.' I knew what he meant because, no matter how perfect the surgical techniques and the post-operative medical care, if the human physiology is not right, the wound or injury just will not heal. However, when it does work, it feels almost miraculous.

I have heard pathologists talk about 'a beautiful wound' in a corpse, one that will never change until putrefaction starts after death, and bodies are refrigerated to slow this process. They mean that the wound is preserving vital forensic evidence in the case of a murder, providing a picture of the direction, force, sharpness or bluntness of the fatal blow for the investigating team. However, the beautiful thing about such a wound for a pathologist is that it is unchanging, whereas in my field, working on live patients, not cadavers, wounds are never beautiful in that way because they are constantly changing and never standing still; the beauty and amazement is in seeing damaged tissue mend, repair and heal, sometimes with barely a mark.

Apart from Tom's other problems, where the original fracture of the mandible had broken through his radiotherapy-damaged skin it had left a hole that would not heal either. It was only small so we initially fixed it in surgery by slightly freshening the edges and then stitching them together, but because of the radiation damage to the skin the edges dissolved and we ended up with a hole on the side of his face bigger than an old fifty-pence piece, through which the titanium metalwork from the fibula flap was now exposed.

We then reconstructed that hole with a flap from his forearm, and because the whole of his lower jaw was already a piece of transplanted fibula, running off the facial arteries and blood vessels on one side of his neck, we had to run the artery and veins for the new flap right round to the blood vessels on the other side of his neck.

Once more the flap was looking good and functioning well at first, but after about fourteen days it started to assume a dusky appearance, which was not a good sign. Again, I suspected that it was a problem with the native tissue surrounding it. We had duplex ultrasound scans of the paddle that showed that blood was still flowing into it and draining from it, but we could not save it and eventually it failed. It was a combination of circumstances that showed us very clearly that the success or failure of a flap is not solely dependent on the blood flow into and out of it; there is something about the bed the flap is sitting on that is also crucial because the flap has to heal on to it and start to acquire a vascular flow through it.

The survival rate for transplanted flaps in some of these difficult cases has now been improved by a development pioneered by a German surgeon using an ECMO (Extra-Corporeal Membrane Oxygenation) machine. This technique was developed for babies born prematurely before thirty weeks, when their underdeveloped lungs won't stay open to exchange gas and instead collapse on themselves. By flooding their lungs with oxygenated fluid rather than air, oxygen is transferred into their bloodstream. In a similar way, instead of attaching a transplanted flap to the blood vessels in the neck, it can be attached to an ECMO machine that will flood the flap with native (the patient's own) oxygenated and anti-coagulated blood. If you do that for a week, so long as the bed the flap is resting on is healthy, the flap will start to stick to its native bed and you can then take away the pedicle connected to the machine and connect it to the patient's own arteries and veins, with a considerably increased chance that it will take.

There was nothing wrong with the pedicle we had used in Tom's flap, but because of the condition of the surrounding tissue, the flap had just fizzled and died. Our next plan to cover this quite sizeable defect was to use part of his pectoralis major, a big sheet of muscle from the chest. We took the flap from the mid-part of Tom's chest but the poor condition of the native tissue on his lower face made us decide to lift up the whole of the pectoralis major and tunnel it up through his neck, while still leaving it attached to the blood vessels in its original site, so that the flap, with a thick pad of muscle attached, was still being supplied by the native blood supply to his chest.

We did it that way because the previous microsurgery had left vulnerable blood vessels running down into the neck from the jaw reconstruction we had already carried out and there was a danger that we might damage them while we were attaching the new flap to the blood vessels in the neck. If so, the original flap from the fibula reconstructing his jaw might well have failed, so we took the safer option of using the largest chest muscle, the pectoralis major, instead. This large sheet of muscle with overlying skin was detached from the right side of the front of his chest, leaving only the blood vessels supplying it attached. It was then rotated up like a propeller into his neck under the skin over his collarbone to provide a solid sheet of healthy muscle and skin to cover his damaged neck.

I told Tom this might affect his golf swing, and that if it improved then credit was due to me. He liked that idea.

So it was defect after defect after defect and pain after pain after pain for poor Tom, but we finally got him healed. After keeping him under close observation until we were sure the procedure had been a success, we were able to send him home to continue his recuperation before returning to hospital to begin planning for the next stage of his rehabilitation. This would involve inserting titanium implants of teeth into his 'new' mandible, eventually enabling us to complete the restoration of his mouth and jaw to their previous appearance and function, so that he could smile, talk and chew food, and life would at last get back to normal for him.

However, Tom then returned to the clinic with a problem. More of the radiation-damaged skin was breaking down over his reconstruction plate. As I write, we are planning to remove the infected plate soon, leaving the new lower jaw and mouth and face skin in place and healed, ready for the next stage for Tom. After two years, and now free of pain, his journey back to health and normal function is still not complete, which only emphasizes the challenges and the lengthy timescales we and our patients often face.

Surgeons like to say that while 'Architects look at their failures, surgeons have to bury theirs'. One of the most famous architects of them all, Frank Lloyd Wright, once countered, 'A doctor can bury his mistakes, but an architect can only advise his clients to plant vines.' An engineer had yet another take on it: 'Doctors bury their mistakes, architects cover theirs with ivy, and engineers write long reports that never see the light of day.'

It is inevitable that not all of my surgical cases will have a happy ending, and in my post-case reflections, even when I have nothing to reproach myself for, I will keep asking myself those same questions, over and over again: 'Did I do everything

I could have? Should I have done more?' As the French surgeon René Leriche wrote in *The Philosophy of Surgery*: 'Every surgeon carries about him a little cemetery, in which from time to time he goes to pray, a cemetery of bitterness and regret, in which he seeks the reason for certain of his failures.' One of the bodies in my cemetery of regrets is that of a lady called Michelle.

She was a bubbly, vivacious barmaid in her early thirties whose first sign of problems came when she began experiencing severe discomfort in her mouth and tongue. Had she had regular dental appointments the problem might have been spotted earlier, but unfortunately she didn't have a dentist and didn't seek medical help until she had reached the point where the pain in her tongue was preventing her from eating. She then phoned NHS Direct for advice. She was sent to her GP and an appointment was at once made for her with the maxillofacial fast-track clinic, and an MRI scan and biopsy were carried out. She was then told she had cancer of the mouth, which is most commonly associated with smokers, heavy drinkers or the over-sixties – none of which applied to Michelle.

Despite the pain of her facial tumour, and the way it was distorting her mouth movement and speech, Michelle smiled through every meeting with us and seemed instantly to trust the team looking after her. To have your patient's trust is a huge privilege, but it can also be the heaviest of burdens. Cancers are not always predictable in the way they affect patients and sometimes you get cancers that are so aggressive right from the kick-off – as was the case with Philip the police constable – that you have a growing uneasy feeling that the disease is not behaving in a way we can ever hope to control, though of course we still have to try our utmost to do so.

Sadly, Michelle's was another such case. Right from the start her cancer seemed to be getting away from us, and, more worrying still, it was changing the way her blood clotted. Cancer cells are essentially normal body cells which are growing out of control and turning on their host. The genome (DNA) in those out-of-control cells is damaged and mutated, which impacts considerably on their immediate environment. For instance, a tumour can grow its own blood supply and the cancer cells can hoodwink the immune system into releasing substances that help them grow rather than subside. A rise in calcium levels or abnormal blood clotting in small blood vessels can also sometimes provide us with unpredictable and worrying signs that can affect the prospects of survival.

We had to remove three-quarters of Michelle's tongue to excise the tumour but performed a free flap to replace it perfectly, using tissue from her stomach wall. However, a blood clot blocked the vein during the operation, and although running at completion, the flap of her tummy muscles rebuilding her tongue and floor of mouth eventually failed. So we repeated the process, once again perfectly, but this time using tissue from her arm. But the same thing happened again, and then again. In total, poor Michelle had to endure nearly twenty hours of surgery over the course of five days before we finally managed to achieve some blood flow. It was still unusually sluggish, so we left two veins attached instead of the normal one, and to further improve the rate of flow we decided to use leech therapy.

Leeches are a natural way to drain blood from human tissue. They are fantastically evolved creatures with a tri-cross of teeth that leave bite marks like a little CND symbol. They secrete anaesthetic so they don't hurt when they bite, and anti-coagulants so the blood supply keeps coming. And they just keep sucking until their stomachs are full, at which point they drop off. Most people react with utter revulsion to the idea of using leeches, but when I told Michelle what the treatment would involve, she just shrugged and said, 'I've never been squeamish, so just do what you have to do to solve the problem.'

They were supplied by a leech farm in South Wales and delivered to the hospital by a bloke on a motorbike. To improve the blood flow through the transplanted flap, Michelle then had to have leeches placed on her tongue four times a day for ten days, but she endured it all without complaint. The leeches were kept in the empty barrel of a 20ml syringe so that they could not escape and fall down into Michelle's throat, trachea or oesophagus. To our delight, the leech therapy worked, and this time the flap did survive, leaving Michelle facing just one more operation to improve her ability to speak and eat.

However, within a few short months she was back to see us again with another lump, a recurrent cancer in the skin on the front of her face. Yet another lump appeared shortly after that, together with a larger one in her neck. The cancer was a hyper-aggressive one that kept getting away from us, and despite attempts to control it with chemotherapy we eventually had to accept that there was nothing more we could do for her.

Michelle had a lovely family, a partner and a seven-year-old daughter. Knowing she was living on borrowed time, she and her partner decided to get married. The local newspaper, the Bradford *Telegraph and Argus*, heard about her desperate situation and launched a campaign to organize the wedding for them. Donations from readers flooded in and the money raised paid for the ceremony and the dress Michelle would wear. The children and teachers at the primary school her daughter attended also organized fund-raising events that added a further £450 to the total. Meanwhile, our technician had been making her a silicone prosthesis to hide the tumours and the holes they formed on her face for her wedding day. It was a more sophisticated version of the ones Harold Gillies had used a century earlier to cover the facial scarring of his patients – just like the mask worn by the fictional Richard Harrow character in *Boardwalk Empire*.

Every fibre of Michelle's being was focused on surviving till her wedding day, and she resisted any suggestion of bringing forward the ceremony, saying, 'I will make it down the aisle one way or another, whether I am walking down or lying down.' Tragically, her boundless courage, determination and optimism were not enough, and she died four weeks before the appointed day, aged just thirty-two. She was buried wearing her wedding dress and the wedding ring that she and her partner had chosen.

I don't often go to patients' funerals – and thankfully there haven't been that many of them – but I felt I needed to go to Michelle's. There was a huge turn-out, and the collection at the end of the service raised a substantial sum of money. Before she died, Michelle had asked that something be put back in to help other cancer sufferers, and her family chose to donate the collection and the remaining money from the newspaper appeal to the surgical team that had looked after her. We used it to set up the Michelle Fuller Head and Neck Research Fund, which helps to sponsor research costs and also produces public information posters. Michelle's name and the fund set up in her memory have appeared on international research presentations in Poznan in Poland, Rhodes in Greece, Toronto, San Francisco and New York. So although she has gone, Michelle continues to inspire us.

Like Michelle, many of my other patients whose own lives have been transformed by surgery have a passionate desire to help others who are facing similar trauma and long-term surgery. Some are dedicated fund-raisers, generating large sums to further our research into earlier detection of cancers, more effective surgical and medical treatments, and improved pre- and post-operative care. Others are willing to act as mentors, sharing experiences and offering hope, solace and consolation to people facing the same traumas that they endured, and a few others have dedicated themselves to raising public awareness and countering some of the misapprehensions, misinformation, fears and prejudices that may prevent people seeking life-saving treatment, sometimes until it is too late.

One of my former patients, Karen, has been a continuing inspiration to me and to all who encounter her. Karen was a schoolteacher who had developed a firm, rubbery nodule on the right side of her face, within the cheek but quite close to her upper wisdom tooth. As a result the initial diagnosis was that the nodule had been caused by trauma to the inside of her cheek from this tooth. Karen was pregnant at the time and she delayed treatment until after the birth of her son, Liam. The lump was then removed by one of the non-cancer surgeons in our team, but unfortunately the wisdom tooth had not been the cause of the nodule. Instead, it proved to be the result of a rare and aggressive form of salivary gland cancer, and when the lump was removed some of the cancerous cells had been left behind.

When Karen came back to the clinic for the results of the excision biopsy the nurses asked her, 'Have you come on your own today, Karen?' As she told me when I saw her soon afterwards, 'I knew right then that this was bad news, and I feared the worst.'

Salivary gland cancer is a 'surgical disease' – a term we use when the only thing that will cure a problem is surgery to remove it (as long as this is possible). Radiotherapy gives unpredictable and generally poor results for this type of cancer, and chemotherapy is not helpful either. So we carried out a very extensive operation, removing the lymph glands from both sides of her neck and carefully dividing the facial skin, muscles and bones, opening up the middle and lower thirds of her face in order to access her cancer and remove it, but maintaining her facial function and hiding the scars. Subsequent tests by the lab showed that the cancer had already spread to one of the glands in her neck, so that part of the operation really had been life-saving. The defect the operation left in her right cheek measured seven centimetres by six and was three centimetres deep, and we reconstructed it using a flap from her non-dominant arm. We then took a skin graft from her tummy to close the arm defect.

Karen recovered well and very quickly, undoubtedly driven by a huge desire to get back to her baby at home. Over and above the standard level of motivation to get this young woman cancer-free and well, we were all particularly energized by the knowledge of that tiny child's need for his mum. She went on to have radiotherapy with Karen Dyker at St James' Infirmary in Leeds, and came out of the other side of it still smiling. Following her recovery from the worst stages of all this treatment, she became a regular visitor at my follow-up clinic, and rarely came empty-handed. Every Easter and Christmas she brought a bag of presents, mostly food and treats, for the department (I had to hide these so I could choose mine before the nurses got to them).

Best of all was the annual Christmas card she gave me, in which I always got another thank you and an update on Liam's progress. Four years after the operation that had saved her life she watched him appear in his primary school's nativity play and then wrote to me, 'I thought that I would never live to see that. Thank you.' The following year's card revealed that he was learning to swim.

On a later visit, Karen, who had been a talented singer before all of this, told me that she had decided to audition for *Britain's Got Talent*. She got through to the round just before the cameras started filming and told her story at each audition. If ever there was proof of the value of function- and face-preserving surgery, that was it. She also came on local radio in Yorkshire with me and spoke with grace and eloquence about her experience when undergoing cancer treatment, and as a cancer survivor. That was very moving for me. Taken out of my professional bubble, I was sitting with someone who was suddenly less a patient than a friend and colleague, helping me to publicize head and neck cancer, and raise money in order to research for better outcomes. Always trying to be an empathetic doctor, I found myself looking at Karen differently as I listened to her speak, and it also gave me a flash of deeper insight into the experience of all our patients, and their families. She talked of the shock of diagnosis and staring into the abyss when the treatment was described, but also of the reassurance she felt through knowing that she had a strong, professional team working to make her better. She also vividly described her fear of not surviving to be a mum for Liam and how that gave her added strength in the dark times when everything seemed impossible.

When he was listening to Karen talking about her treatment and the extent of her facial surgery, the host of the radio show just kept staring at her face and repeating, 'You would not know! You really would not know!' I was an observer now, not a professional carer in the pilot seat driving fast towards a cure – just another person sitting next to Karen, and hearing this with different ears, feeling the impact of all that she had endured to survive for her son. And as I observed I realized that my 'professional shield' would need constant adjustment to allow me to be empathetic and compassionate but still a functional, solid, professional surgeon. Karen and I were in a fairly stressful live radio interview together, working to a common aim, and I saw her perform superbly for the cause, speaking so clearly, alive and looking so well because of the efforts of our team. I am still sometimes amazed by all that has been gained in the last century, by the striving of others before me, handing down skills that I have been able to learn and use with the team and other surgeons (Dave Sutton in this case), so that I could be sitting there next to Karen, a true survivor and a wonderful mother, speaking for us on live broadcast media.

Over the years I've been privileged to be able to develop my skills as a maxillofacial surgeon. I've also become the leader of a ground-breaking clinical research team. When I apply for major research grant funding there is always a section on the forms for a lay explanation of the planned work and what it will bring. It is an essential part of the process, because if there has been no consultation with members of the public, major awarding bodies will not give funding at all. Karen has helped me in that process too by being a proofreader for me for a number of these applications. As a schoolteacher, she has a fearsome red pen, and her input has been hugely significant in fixing my sometimes jargon-laden and opaque medical terminology – though at one stage I did have to ask her if I could have an occasional gold star as well as all the red pen marks . . .

Any application for funding has to be preceded by the involvement of patients and carers. We do this by organizing meetings where I present our research plans and record the feedback. I have always particularly enjoyed these events, probably because it is a different level of engagement with the people our team cares for. I have a policy for these meetings of using exactly the same slides as I do for presentations to scientists and research surgeons, but I put the information in layman's terms, not to patronize the audience but because the dialogue between surgeons and scientists is often so riddled with jargon and acronyms that it is almost impossible to follow if you are unfamiliar with medical terminology.

When asked about the merits of our research, the response from members of the public has often been, 'Of course it's a good idea – are you mad? Why hasn't someone done this already?' But there have also been some sharp insights into the proposed logistics. I think my enjoyment of these events comes from the sharing of high-level, cutting-edge science with people under my care. I want them to know the heights we are trying to reach to improve early detection of cancers and minimize harm, while still achieving a cure and planning for survival after cancer. There is no doubt that people regard the medical team differently after these events, and they are a vital part of the process of funding our clinical research.

Clearly the patients are also given a high degree of autonomy when they are offered the opportunity to participate in our research work. Despite our careful consideration for them and compassionate delivery of information, a patient with a cancer diagnosis has only two choices: go with the treatment or refuse it. The former often seems like stepping on to a rollercoaster and holding on to the bars, white-knuckled, until it stops, but the latter is not to get on at all and face the consequences. This may be why our discussions are so often well received by our patients, and go along these lines:

'Will this help me, doctor?'

'I don't know, that's why we are running the trial.'

'OK. Well, will it help someone else?'

'Definitely.'

'Great! Where do I sign?'

The randomized controlled clinical trial is the gold standard to prove that something works, and I have been involved in a number of them over the years. My biggest success to date is the Lugol's Iodine Head and Neck Cancer Surgery (LIHNCS) trial, using potassium iodide to identify normal cells at the edges of cancers, the purpose being that cells that don't turn brown are pre-cancer cells and can be taken away at the same time as the cancer, which means that we won't be leaving behind a ticking time bomb. A total of 419 patients took part in twenty-four centres in the UK. Less than 10 per cent of patients asked if they wished to take part turned down the chance – proof positive of the altruism of the majority of the British population. However, not all clinical trials are of equal value and there is a danger of them being used unnecessarily, consuming scarce resources and the time of skilled researchers to provide proof of something that a little thought would have shown was pretty much self-evident anyway.

I first met Gordon Smith, now Professor of Obstetrics at Cambridge, when he was a senior registrar in Glasgow; in fact he delivered our son James. Although discussion on that day was limited, I knew he was a researcher of some talent. Some years later, Gordon and his team published, in the Christmas edition of the *British Medical Journal*, a gentle mickey-take of some of the fanatical evangelists of evidence-based medicine, by describing the set-up of a proper randomized controlled trial to assess the efficacy of using a parachute when jumping from an aeroplane.

The research methodology would be straightforward. Two groups would be randomized: those with a parachute and those with no parachute. The results might appear to be self-evident, but might not be quite so clear cut, because some of the parachutes might not open and some people with parachutes might be strangled by the cords. By the same token, some of the people without parachutes might be lucky enough to land on a hayrick or in a snowdrift that would cushion their fall and enable them to survive. So would the trial actually prove that a parachute is necessary and jumping without one really dangerous? Furthermore, to ensure a fully randomized trial, having carried out the first test all the survivors would have to be crossed over to the opposite group and the experiment repeated . . .

That scenario was deliberately absurd, but some genuine randomized controlled trials appear to be only slightly less ridiculous. Although tongue in cheek, the article highlighted the point that if there is a new method of treatment versus an old one and there's no certainty about which might work better, by all means do the trial, but if there is a clear scientific, mechanistic explanation for why something should work (e.g. air resistance against parachute silk), you really don't need to have a clinical trial to prove it.

14

ONE OF THE most difficult and contentious issues in modern medicine is how to predict who is capable of withstanding treatment. Accompanied by one of his daughters, Malcolm sat calmly and quietly waiting to see me, having already been seen by one of our department's associate specialists who did not appear to have had the benefit of a course on how to break bad news to patients, because he had been rather direct in his transmission of information about Malcolm's condition – oral cancer – both to him and to his daughter.

When I met him, Malcolm was neatly dressed and said very little at first. His facial appearance was that of a man who had smoked heavily for many years, while his florid complexion and the broken capillaries and veins in his nose and face also suggested that he was far from a stranger to alcohol. So after I had introduced myself and spent a few minutes talking to him to establish a degree of trust between us, I asked him about his smoking and drinking. In response, he admitted to drinking a moderate amount of alcohol each day and also said that he had smoked thirty cigarettes a day for fifty years. That would have to change, and I explained the need for him to stop smoking before his treatment began. He told me, with evident steely determination, that he felt certain he could do this.

His medical problem was a lump in the floor of his mouth which was firm and becoming so painful that he was unable to wear his lower denture. After enduring the discomfort for a while he had eventually sought an appointment with his general practitioner, who had immediately sent him to see us under the 'two-week, fast-track, could this be cancer?' system that we were operating in cooperation with the GPs in our area. He was scanned that very morning and a biopsy was arranged. The scan showed that the cancer itself was still small and confined to the floor of his mouth, but it also revealed a second lump at the back of his nasopharynx – the part of the nose that connects to the throat. That would require further investigation before we could decide how best to treat the original tumour.

The next time I met him he was accompanied by both of his daughters, and I noted that the one I had not met previously was wearing a nurse's uniform. There was a more detailed discussion between all of us and she explained that her father had great difficulty in 'getting going' until lunchtime because of difficulties with his chest and shortness of breath. However, when I asked him 'Malcolm, could you climb a flight of stairs?', he straightened in his chair, looked me straight in the eye and said, 'Of course I could.' Despite his apparent confidence, I had my doubts.

As mandated by the decision of our surgical team, I explained that, before removing the tumour from his mouth, we would need to learn more about the nature of the lump at the back of his nose. I was hopeful that this was merely a benign cyst or simply a part of his normal anatomy, but we could not proceed to treat his tumour until we knew for sure.

There had also been some concern over his fitness for the operation. In general, with some reservations, the surgical team felt that he would be capable of undergoing the surgery, but one of the anaesthetic consultants did express his concern that our patient might not be physically strong enough to survive the procedure. In the light of that, the short general anaesthetic he would need to undergo to enable us to investigate the lump at the back of his nose would be a helpful indicator for us of how capable he would be of withstanding a seven- or eight-hour procedure to cure his tumour.

Three days later, Malcolm was admitted to the ward and signed his consent for an examination under anaesthesia and a biopsy of the mass at the back of his nasopharynx. The operation, using a fibre-optic scope, was complicated because of a deviation in his nasal septum – the bone and cartilage that separates the two nostrils. Most people have some minor deviation, but Malcolm's was so crooked that it was indicative of serious damage from physical trauma in the past. It was causing some obstruction of his breathing but it also prevented me from passing any surgical instruments up his nose. That caused obvious difficulties in terms of accessing the lump at the back of his nose, but in the end I was able to pass my surgical gloved hand around the back of his soft palate and manipulate the lump directly with my finger.

I then asked the nursing sister to find me some finer rigid forceps and I was able to pass these, albeit with some difficulty, down the left-hand side of his nose to meet my finger. I could now clearly feel the new lump, which was smooth in outline, and although it was quite solid to the touch it appeared unlikely to be a cancer deposit representing a new tumour.

Bleeding from the biopsy was excessive at first and I controlled the warm, gushing blood with firm pressure from my surgical finger and a swab. We then placed a haemostatic gel in the very back of the nose, and some Merocel packs that we use after rhinoplasty (also known as 'a nose job') on the left and right nostrils. These allow air to pass through but apply constant pressure to the nasal septum, stemming blood flow. Once the bleeding had stopped, I applied some local anaesthetic to the back of his throat and nasopharynx, to make sure he woke up feeling comfortable and with no further bleeding.

Malcolm returned to the ward via the recovery area, but very soon afterwards he became short of breath and normal respiration became problematic. In the days that followed, we learned that the cyst at the back of his nose had been benign and was of no consequence, having been completely treated by removing it. We were then left with the plan to excise his tumour, remove the glands from his neck and reconstruct the defect in his mouth with a microsurgery free flap. It would be an intricate, complex procedure that would be life-saving for him, but routine, though still demanding, for our team.

I went to see Malcolm on the ward and found him sitting up in bed, breathing supplementary oxygen and coughing loudly. The physiotherapy team had seen him and given him some breathing exercises, as well as massaging his chest in an effort to ease his respiratory problems, but his inflammatory markers and observations in general were deteriorating, indicating that a chest infection was developing.

Despite the best efforts of twenty-first-century surgical and medical care, his chest just grew worse and he eventually developed a full lower respiratory tract infection, or pneumonia. Even using ventilator support, antibiotics and physiotherapy we were unable to stave off the continuing deterioration in Malcolm's health and he eventually died of pneumonia, secondary to his cancer, before we were able to start to cure him of it.

His case highlighted the difficulties in assessing whether patients who are old and/or in poor health are sufficiently robust to survive the treatment required to cure their cancers. Modern medicine has developed a number of different scoring systems to try to help predict the likely outcomes when patients such as Malcolm are ill and, working with our head and neck anaesthetic team, we are also constantly searching for indicators that will help us to make the right decisions for our patients. But whatever system of evaluation we adopt, years of experience teach us that in some patients, the emergence of a lump can be a 'pre-terminal event'.

It's like the situation when an elderly lady is found having fallen at home and fractured her hip. The novice surgeon will focus on the hip fracture and rush to operate immediately, which of course is the right treatment for the injury; but as he or she becomes more experienced, the realization may dawn that the reason the lady fell over was because of a general deterioration of the organs, glands, tissues and cells that control body temperature, fluid composition, blood sugar, blood pressure, etc., so the fall was a pre-terminal event.

In such cases, whatever medical or surgical treatment we try to offer will make no difference; we can repair the effects of that particular trauma but we can do nothing about the general health failure that led to it, and the patient will not recover. Such cases, with their inevitably depressing conclusions, can lead the assessing surgical and anaesthetic teams to feel more like helpless bystanders than caring physicians. It is a constant background to what we do, though, because the number of patients in this kind of situation is already high and rising in line with the general increase in life expectancy.

Assessing the preferred treatment options and their likely outcomes also has to be balanced with the overall perception of the needs of an individual patient. This was emphasized by the case of Montgomery v. Lanarkshire Health Board. In 1999, a diabetic mother gave birth to a baby with severe disabilities (cerebral palsy) because of difficulties during the birth that arose when she was delivered in the normal vaginal fashion rather than by Caesarean section. Diabetic mothers are much more likely to have larger-than-average babies and such cases carry a 10 per cent risk that the baby will suffer shoulder dystocia – dislocation of the shoulder – and difficulties being born naturally because they are simply too large to pass through the mother's pelvic opening. Although the patient had expressed her concerns about having a normal vaginal delivery, the policy of the consultant obstetrician and gynaecologist was not to tell any diabetic women about the possibility of shoulder dystocia, because she believed that the risk of serious problems for the baby was very small, and if told about shoulder dystocia, women patients would inevitably opt for a Caesarean. After problems with the birth did arise, resulting in the baby being born with severe disabilities, the consultant was accused of neglect.

The case went all the way to the Supreme Court, which ruled that it was a mistake to view patients as uninformed and incapable of understanding medical matters or wholly dependent on information from doctors in order to reach decisions. Patients of sound mind were entitled to decide which of the available treatments to accept, and the patient's consent had to be obtained before any treatment involving 'interfering with her bodily integrity' was undertaken. In this case, the treatment involved a 'substantial risk of grave adverse consequences', and the court concluded that a patient's right to decide whether to assent to a particular course of treatment was 'so obvious that no prudent doctor could fail to warn of the risk'. Irrespective of the slight risk of serious disabilities to the baby arising from a natural birth, the Supreme Court found that shoulder dystocia itself was 'a major obstetric emergency; the contrast to the tiny risk to the woman and baby involved in an elective Caesarean is stark'.

The implication for other doctors and surgeons seems to be that, although the treating team had done almost everything correctly in purely medical terms, when obtaining the consent of a patient for any procedure there is a clear need to establish the level of importance that he or she places on any particular outcome. That of course would extend to the risk of death, and given the certainty of an unpleasant death from cancer, any patient given even a 50 per cent chance of surviving a procedure may well wish to take their chances in the hope of survival.

So decisions must be taken as the result of dialogue with patients, to establish how much importance they place on a particular complication, which can vary dramatically. An operation to remove part of the thyroid gland, which may produce a hoarse voice, can have a completely different impact on a radio or television newsreader compared to someone who works quietly as a librarian. Both clearly require good vocal function in order to live in our modern society, but for one their entire livelihood depends on it.

The process of decision-making on whether or not to offer surgery is growing more sophisticated, and so too is the technology at a surgeon's disposal. One example we have already met in earlier chapters – the harmonic scalpel, which looks like a pair of surgical scissors with a Stormtrooper upgrade outfit, attached to a device that generates energy and sets an active blade vibrating faster than audible sounds. When human tissue is squashed gently between this and the other (passive) blade it divides the tissue but also seals the blood vessels on either side of it, which is particularly useful for areas prone to excessive bleeding, like the tongue.

We also have two kinds of diathermy electrosurgery, using high-frequency shortwave electric current to generate deep heat in body tissues. The bipolar version passes electricity at high frequency between the ends of forceps, which burn and seal the tissue in between. The current in the monopolar model passes from the tip of the instrument to a paddle on the patient's thigh. It only develops heat at the tip of the instrument in the surgeon's hand, but cannot be used if the patient has any metalwork (which would act as a conductor) in his body.

High-resolution CT scans have also enabled us to produce 3D-printed models of patients' skulls and facial bones, improving pre-operative planning. The industrial use of CAD/CAM (Computer Aided Design/Computer Aided Manufacturing) to produce precision components has also led to the development of patient-specific medical implants, while using materials such as titanium and PEEK (polyether ether ketone – a colourless, organic, thermoplastic polymer) allows us to recreate the patient's original facial features. The same technology has enabled us to make cutting guides that produce more accurate harvesting and moulding of the free flaps used to reconstruct the patient's facial features.

Although such new technology means that our ability to make effective surgical interventions continues to improve, we still require the purely human qualities of experience, wisdom and strength to help us know when to make the decision *not* to operate on a patient when in other circumstances he would benefit from surgery.

The balance of benefit over risk must always be clearly understood to be in the patient's favour, but that may require an even more developed discussion about their treatment, survival chances and preferences. Survey after survey demonstrates that people would most prefer to die quietly and comfortably in their own homes, yet the majority of us still do not do so. Perhaps the least dignified death of all is in a hospital in the middle of a flurry of activity and the mess of body fluids and smells and sounds of a cardiac arrest call at four o'clock in the morning, yet that is the fate that awaits all too many of our patients.

Clinicians treating cancer patients can feel that their choice is often either to condemn them to death from cancer, which is never easy or pleasant, or to death on the operating table or very soon afterwards, in an attempt to avert the former fate. It is also often apparent in our discussions that none of the people on our side of the operating table has ever had to face such a decision. Once again we must evaluate very carefully our patients' wishes and how that might affect our attitude to the treatment of men like Malcolm, or on the other hand another patient of mine, Mrs White. Despite being ninety-six years old, she was in such excellent physical condition that she had a tumour excised from her mouth and a transplant of a free flap to repair the ensuing defect, and not only did she survive the operation, she lived for another ten years after it. Her sister had lived to 105 at the time she presented, so the clue regarding good genes and survival was clear.

By contrast, Malcolm's case was an example of what can be a very serious issue: co-morbidities – one or more additional diseases or disorders co-existing with a primary one. In some cancer patients co-morbidities are nothing short of startling. Although the vast majority of the patients I now see in Glasgow tend to be in reasonable health, take some exercise, eat a fairly sensible diet and are not addicted to nicotine, alcohol or Class A drugs, there are a few who are a real challenge, not just to the medical profession but to society as a whole.

We can't cure every patient, though that is always our aim, but they have a role to play too; yet a surprisingly large number seem unwilling to take the necessary steps to improve their own health. I've asked people to reduce their drinking or smoking or preferably stop altogether, and been given a flat 'No'.

A recent patient had a pre-cancer patch in his mouth that we were going to stain and remove with lasers. He was scheduled to be the penultimate operation on my last day before my holidays but as soon as he was anaesthetized he became unwell with heart and chest issues that, like his pre-cancerous patch, were due to his refusal to cut down or stop smoking. So not only had he caused himself distress and created complications for the surgical team, his treatment took so long that by the time we had finished with him it was also too late to begin operating on the last patient of the day. So his stubborn refusal to take the step that would have improved his health and probably lengthened his life also meant that another patient's treatment had to be postponed with potentially serious implications for him.

Lack of exercise, poor diet, heavy smoking and excessive drinking mean many patients are in a very poor state of health prior to treatment. As a result, it is often questionable whether they will be able to survive the prolonged anaesthesia and surgery, not to mention the post-operative recovery period necessary to cure their cancer, but frustratingly for the surgical team there is no good objective test to which we can refer to establish whether such patients are likely to survive their treatment. No test can accurately predict whether a particular individual will do well or badly, nor what sort of complications they are likely to develop.

The West of Scotland team is absolutely forensic in terms of examining the complications patients can develop during and after their treatment; everything is meticulously documented, and every month the previous four weeks' cases are discussed in detail. When I began working with that system it was a revelation to me, because no other hospital or trust is going into fine details like that, but they really should be because learning the lessons from those complications should help to ensure better patient outcomes in the future.

Sometimes you have to accept that if you operate to remove a cancer and reconstruct the defect in the patient by transplanting a free flap from elsewhere in the body, the consequences of that, together with the side-effects of the treatment – almost always involving what are essentially lung injuries and chest infections – may be not a cure but either the death of the patient or at the very least a prolonged stay in an Intensive Care Unit. If the patient does not survive, their demise then becomes our fault, and it is one of those classic situations where we are damned if we do and damned if we don't. We take the blame if we don't treat them and they then survive a long time before dying a horrible death from cancer, but we are also blamed if we decide to go ahead with the treatment but they then die in hospital soon afterwards.

There is a wider ethical debate about how we should deal with patients whose lifestyles have either caused, or at the least contributed substantially to, the health problems they have developed, but it is a debate that the government and British society as a whole should be engaging with, not just the medical profession. The million-dollar question is, how much of the NHS's ever-dwindling pool of time, workforce and resources should we actually be allocating to patients whose lifestyles mean that they are effectively suffering from self-inflicted wounds?

Some would argue that if patients are unwilling to modify and improve their lifestyles we should not be allocating increasingly scarce resources to them that would be better devoted to patients with a better chance of successful long-term outcomes. That is not a view most doctors would be comfortable holding. The issue poses an emotive and horribly controversial ethical dilemma – a proper can of worms – that society as a whole has yet to address.

Poor lifestyles are often linked to social deprivation, of course, and one of the consequences of that is that hospitals sited in regions of high unemployment, low incomes and poor housing, with all the attendant social problems, may appear to be less clinically effective than hospitals in more affluent areas. For example, if I am carrying out operations on hard-drinking, heavy-smoking Glaswegians who also have a poor diet, while another surgeon is doing operations on the kind of self-referred Home Counties people who tend to arrive at a hospital like the Royal Marsden in London, the latter's patient outcomes are inevitably going to be better than mine, but that's because the substrates he is starting from are quite different.

In an attempt to address that problem, a Clinical Fellow in London, David Tighe, got involved with other surgeons and scientists including Jeremy McMahon in Glasgow and started trying to factor in co-morbidities and other aspects about patients and their cancers in different hospitals and regions around the country that will predict their probable outcomes. Using their methods, when the issue of Home Counties affluence, for example, was factored into the statistics of the Royal Marsden in London, which had the best patient outcomes overall, it corrected away from the mean, whereas when the social factors governing the base populations of hospitals in more deprived regions were added to the mix, they all corrected towards it.

Glasgow took a massive leap towards the mean, but still remained an outlier compared to the majority of other hospitals. But I think that is not just because of the poverty, poor diet and social and lifestyle problems in parts of the Glasgow hospitals' catchment area, though they certainly do exist. As I mentioned earlier, the Maxillofacial/Head and Neck team in Glasgow forensically records every complication its patients suffer, right down to a stitch abscess, which in my experience no other hospitals do. So in this preliminary work Glasgow is effectively being penalized in its comparative statistics because of its meticulous care in documenting its patients' treatment and any ensuing complications.

Furthermore, things that are factored in as complications in one unit may not be regarded as such in another, leading to a false comparison between them, and regrettably, the way that the statistics are compiled may also influence the way a case is treated. For example, a blood transfusion is not regarded as a complication if it is carried out at the time of an operation, but if it becomes necessary after the operation then it is recorded as a complication, affecting that unit's statistics, so there may be a temptation to give a transfusion at the time of the operation, even if it is not clearly necessary, just to avoid doing one subsequently and having it recorded in the figures.

Having an unnecessary blood transfusion matters because a blood transfusion is immuno-suppressive, and when you control for factors like the level of blood loss and the size of the operation, cancer patients more frequently get a recurrence of their cancer if they have had a transfusion. That is still the case even though for transfusions we now use 'packed cells' that have been depleted of lymphocytes – the white blood cells and antibodies. Patients only need red blood cells in transfusions, and as long as they are matched to the patient by blood type, they don't provoke an immune response. As a result, blood for transfusion is routinely filtered to remove as many of the white blood cells, proteins and antibodies as possible. However, it is simply not possible to remove absolutely every trace of the blood donor's white cells and antibodies, and transfused blood therefore still contains factors from the donor that will trigger an immune response in the recipient of the blood. The more complex the cancer that we are treating, the greater the quantity of transfused blood the patient is likely to need, and therefore the stronger the immune response triggered in the patient, diverting some of their own natural defences away from battling the cancer to fighting the factors within the transfused blood.

Quite apart from all this, we also ought to be asking ourselves if the obsession with collecting and analysing quite so many statistics is really the way we ought to be going, since it may well cause surgeons and doctors to pause and ponder the potential impact on their figures before embarking on a particular course of treatment. In the old days one or two surgeons might have escaped proper scrutiny or the consequences of mistakes they had made in a way that would not be possible now, but on the other side of the coin, nor did any of them have to spend their time worrying how it might look on their stats if there were complications in a particular procedure. Instead they were free to concentrate their entire attention on what was best for the patient. I hope and believe that the needs of the patient remain uppermost in the minds of every medical professional, but I would be more confident of that if there were less stress on the sort of performance statistics and league tables that have already blighted our educational system.

If the level of resource required to collect high-quality data was made available and interacted with the clinical teams in the same way as our clinical research trials, surgeons would have more confidence in the data. A large randomized clinical trial will cost in the region of £500,000 to run over a five- to seven-year period. Yet often we are asked to complete assessment projects on outcomes by which we will be measured, compared, praised or damned with no extra funding at all. By any yardstick that cannot be the way to move forward.

15

THE ABILITY TO restore facial features has been sought throughout the history of modern medicine and surgery. By first conquering excessive blood loss and then by managing anaesthesia, together with understanding how to control infection, doctors came to understand how our immune system will both protect us and reject foreign material, or 'non-self-tissue', applied to the human physiology. Developments in microvascular free tissue transfer have allowed us to transplant body parts from the arms, legs, chest, abdomen, back and pelvis into the human face, to restore a patient's looks and their ability to speak, eat and swallow.

Another solution may be to repair the facial structures but conceal the remaining damage behind a prosthetic mask. Perhaps the most moving example of this comes not from my casebook but from that of a good friend, the American maxillo-facial surgeon Dr Eric Dierks. Eric's patient, Chrissy, was a beautiful, blue-eyed, blonde sixteen-year-old who had gone somewhat astray in her life and was in the getaway car when some other teenagers robbed a country store and gun shop, escaping with fifteen stolen guns. A few weeks after the robbery they were drinking with a dozen friends when one of them began messing around with a stolen twelve-bore shotgun. A second later the gun went off at point-blank range, blasting through her face from below her right eye to the hairline on her left temple.

Chrissy could easily have died from her injuries and blood loss. Trauma surgery saved her life, but there was now a gaping hole where her nose, eyes, cheeks and most of her mouth had been, and she was blind. As Eric said, 'I've not seen anything quite so severe, where the patient lived.'

When she had recovered, Eric and his team began the reconstruction. They used pieces of her fibula and titanium plates to construct new cheekbones and bridge the missing part of her face, then covered it with a free flap of flesh and skin from her leg, but they could not restore her sight, nor immediately rectify the 'caved-in' look of the middle part of her face. She had to breathe through her mouth because her nose no longer existed.

After emerging from that first lengthy spell in hospital, Chrissy took stock of her situation. 'When I realized what had happened to me, I knew I could either sit back and have a "pity party" or figure out what to do with the rest of my life.' Resolving to make the best of her situation, she went back to High School, graduated with straight As and, wearing an elegant white mask, went to her High School Prom on the arm of a family friend.

For the next decade Chrissy only went out with an oversize black sleep-mask covering her face, and even though she was blind, she could sense and sometimes hear that people were staring at her and speculating about what had happened to her. While going to classes for the blind, she met and fell in love with Geoff Dilger, who had also been blinded at the age of sixteen. They moved in together, and seven years later Chrissy gave birth to a son. She had almost resigned herself to living with her deformity for the rest of her life, but the birth of her child made her determined that he would not grow up looking at his mother's ravaged face. That was one of the prime factors that persuaded her to seek further treatment.

However, Eric's desire to give Chrissy a face transplant or embark on a series of surgical procedures to build her a new one was hampered by the state Medicaid's refusal to cover the cost of it. Eric then decided to construct a prosthesis. 'A face transplant would still not give her seeing eyes, nor would it give her mobile eyelids and lashes,' he said at the time. 'There's no way we can return that to her, and the prosthesis will look as good and possibly better than a face transplant.' But Medicaid wouldn't pay for a prosthesis either, continuing to insist it was a purely cosmetic procedure, much to the anger of her surgeons. Eric and two prosthodontists then agreed to carry out the work for nothing, while the hospital covered the additional costs of her treatment and a dental company donated the implants.

The first priority was to remove some damaged tissue and trim the implants from the fibula that had been used to reconstruct the structures of her mid-face, and then open a new nasal cavity in Chrissy's face so that she no longer had to breathe through her mouth. After waiting a few months for that to heal, Eric then drilled eight titanium dental implants into her facial bones that would act as 'anchors' for the prosthetic mask. Another four months elapsed while they waited for the implants to fuse with the bones, then came the final stage, the creation of the prosthetic mask.

In a process that was part science, part art, and working from photographs of Chrissy before the gunshot incident but allowing for the ageing process over the intervening decade, the prosthodontists made a plaster cast of her existing face. They then poured skin-toned silicone into it to form the basic prosthesis. It was hand-painted to mimic the natural look of human skin and, in consultation with Chrissy and using her favourite brand, make-up was then applied. The whole mask was then baked so that the skin tones and make-up became permanent. The edges of the prosthesis were made wafer-thin and almost translucent, allowing it to blend as seamlessly as possible with Chrissy's natural facial skin. Acrylic eyes were inserted and carefully positioned so that her gaze looked natural, and false eyelashes were individually inserted with tweezers.

The finished mask was attached to Chrissy's face using magnets connected to the dental implants, allowing it to be snapped on and off with ease. When she unveiled her prosthesis to her family for the first time, her mother burst into tears of happiness.

'When anyone finds out how I went blind,' Chrissy says, 'their first comment ninety-nine per cent of the time is to say "I'm sorry." And my response to that is: "I'm not. I lived. There's nothing to be sorry about living after something like that. Don't be sorry for me, be happy for me. Be proud of the fact that I've gone on with my life." '*

Chrissy now has her mask, but in other cases where a patient's face is so comprehensively and extensively damaged, only by replacing all of the soft tissues can we produce a result that will eliminate the visible evidence of their horrific facial trauma, pain and suffering.

Facial transplantation is a very new development. It first emerged in popular culture in the 1960 cult horror film *Les Yeux Sans Visages*, but, as so often in the past, life has now imitated art,

---

* Additional quotations taken from Don Colburn's articles in *The Oregonian* newspaper and Ashleigh Banfield's reporting for ABC News.

and in recent years science fiction has turned into science fact with the concept of surgically transplanting a human face becoming first a ground-breaking reality, and then a routine procedure.

The first face transplant in the world was carried out in November 2005 by a French maxillofacial surgeon, Bernard Devauchelle. In May of that year his patient, Isabelle Dinoire, in an apparent attempt to take her own life – though that interpretation has been disputed by members of her family – had locked herself in a room in her apartment and taken an overdose of medication. 'After a very upsetting week, with many personal problems,' she later said, 'I took some pills to forget . . . I fainted and fell on the ground, hitting a piece of furniture.'

Her pet Labrador dog had been trapped in the room with her and, perhaps in a desperate attempt to revive the unconscious Isabelle, the dog began scratching and clawing at her, and pulling and biting the mid-part of her face. Whether or not Isabelle intended to commit suicide, by the time she regained consciousness in the room some time later, the dog had bitten and clawed off a large amount of the facial soft tissue from her nose, upper lip, mouth and cheeks.

Isabelle later described waking up in a pool of blood with the dog by her side. At first unaware of the state of her face – the residual effects of the drugs she had swallowed would have masked most of the pain – she attempted to light a cigarette, but found it strange that she was unable to hold it in her mouth. She then phoned her two teenage daughters, who had been spending the night at their grandmother's house, and asked them if they wanted to take the dog for a walk.

The elder daughter thought that her mother's voice 'sounded

funny', but only when they returned home and let themselves into the darkened room did they realize that she was seriously injured. They found the floor covered in blood and their mother's face completely unrecognizable. One can only imagine the horror and distress the sight must have engendered in them.

It was only when Isabelle caught sight of her altered facial appearance in the mirror that she realized what had happened. She stated in subsequent interviews that at first 'I couldn't even begin to imagine it was my face and my blood, or that the dog had chewed my face'.

The French authorities immediately put the dog down, much to Isabelle's distress. Despite her injuries, she did not blame her pet for the incident and was 'heartbroken' at its fate. She kept a picture of the dog by her hospital bedside.

After preliminary treatment for her injuries, in the months following her release from hospital Isabelle only went out in public with a mask covering the lower half of her face and, lacking lips, she had great difficulty in speaking and making herself understood. When her medical team, which also included Jean-Michel Dubernard, another maxillofacial surgeon, and Benoît Lengelé, a Belgian plastic surgeon, surveyed the damage to her face they had immediately ruled out the possibility of reconstruction by standard means – a free flap transfer of her own tissue from elsewhere in her body – and had begun attempts to find a donor for the world's first face transplant.

The search occupied several months, but towards the end of 2005 a suitable donor was at last found. After an operation lasting fifteen hours, the team of surgeons succeeded in restoring

Isabelle's facial appearance to something like normality, albeit with a completely different face from her own, by transplanting the entire nose, cheeks, upper and lower lips and other soft tissue from the deceased donor, another French woman who, in a strange coincidence, had also attempted to commit suicide, in her case successfully. As Isabelle remarked in her own later account of her ordeal, that gave her 'a feeling of sisterhood' with the unwitting donor of her new face.

When she awoke in the hospital's Intensive Care Unit following the operation, Isabelle was given a mirror and allowed to see her new face for the first time. She scribbled the word 'Merci' on a message board that a nurse held for her, and then 'she cried and cried' – but, as one of her medical team commented, 'everyone in the room cried'. As Isabelle later said, 'From the first time I saw myself in the mirror after the operation I knew it was a victory. It didn't look that good because of all the bandages, but I had a nose, I had a mouth, it was fantastic. I could see in the eyes of the nurses that it was a success.'

In 2012, seven years after the operation, Isabelle described in an interview how she had managed to cope both with the stares of people she passed in the street and the unfulfilled yearning that she felt to meet the family of the woman whose face she now had. She stated in the interview that 'the most difficult thing is to find myself again as the person I was, with the face I had before the accident. But I know that's not possible . . . When I look in the mirror, I see a mixture of the two of us. The donor is always with me – she saved my life.'

Long after the operation Isabelle continued to be pursued by the media and was often harassed by passers-by and curious onlookers. She lived in a small town in northern France and everyone there knew what had happened to her. She talked of children laughing at her in the street and people pointing and staring. As a result she spent many months virtually confined to her house, feeling unable to leave the sanctuary of her own home. There was also a long process of personal adjustment, simply getting used to the new face. As time passed, people still recognized her and stared, but by then she felt able to stare back without being distressed by it, until they looked away.

The news of the first successful face transplant provoked an immediate, fierce debate about the ethics of the procedure. Carrying out a transplant for a non-fatal condition bore a significant risk, because approximately one-third of all major transplants end in the patient's death, either because the body's natural defences reject the transplant or because the immuno-suppressant drugs used to prevent that leave the body prey to cancers and other fatal diseases. Some critics also hinted, without being brave enough to expose themselves to the risk of legal proceedings by openly stating it, that the surgeons might have been motivated more by the fame attendant on carrying out the first face transplant – racing to complete the first procedure in competition with a team of surgeons in the United States who were also looking for a suitable donor and recipient – than by concerns for their patient's welfare.

As with other transplant patients, the health risks to Isabelle did not end with the operation. Even when such surgery is successful, patients are condemned to a lifetime of taking anti-rejection drugs with dangerous and, in the medium to long term, potentially fatal side-effects. There is also a very long recuperative period and, in Isabelle's case, the additional psychological problems that came with seeing someone else's face looking back at her from the mirror. Critics pointed to the mental instability implicit in her suicide attempt and condemned what they saw as a rush to carry out transplant surgery without first fully assessing whether more conventional reconstruction techniques might not have been just as effective and less traumatic – psychologically, if not physically – for this particular patient.

However, as Dr Dubernard stated, 'Once I had seen Isabelle's disfigured face, no more needed to be said.' 'Full-face' transplants are now increasingly frequent. In August 2015 surgeons at New York University's Langone Medical Center, led by Eduardo Rodriguez, carried out the most extensive facial transplant yet. One hundred surgeons and medical staff working in two teams over a period of twenty-six hours successfully transplanted the face of David Rodebaugh, a twenty-six-year-old who had been left in a permanent vegetative state after a cycling accident, on to David Hardison, a forty-one-year-old former fireman and father of five children who had suffered appalling injuries when a burning roof collapsed on him, melting his breathing mask on to his face. Rodebaugh's mother gave her blessing to the procedure, saying that her son had been 'born a miracle . . . [and now] the miracle of David will live on'.

Hardison had endured fourteen years of absolute misery before the transplant, including no fewer than seventy-one operations, and had become addicted to the painkillers prescribed to help him cope with the agony caused whenever he moved any part of his hideously scarred face. He was almost in a situation where 'the pain of living is worse than death'.* On the rare occasions he went out in public, he wore a baseball cap, dark glasses and prosthetic ears to hide his injuries and avoid

---

* From Selma Lagerlöf, *Antikrists Mirakler* ['The Miracles of Antichrist'], 1899.

having to witness the discomfort, aversion or even terror in the faces of people he encountered. His transplant was third-time-lucky for him: he had previously been offered two other faces. The first was that of a Hispanic man whose family then changed their minds and withdrew their consent, and the second was that of a woman, which Hardison himself turned down.

Arguments about the morality of carrying out face transplants have continued, with one bioethicist remarking, 'I'm not against face transplants but I think we are travelling at too fast a speed. People may ask what could be worse than living with a distorted face. Well, you could be dead.' However, those who question the ethics of such operations might bear in mind David Hardison's comments about his appearance before his transplant, published in *New York Magazine*. 'Kids ran screaming and crying when they saw me,' he said. 'There are things worse than dying.'

Criticisms were also brushed aside by the surgeons who operated on Isabelle Dinoire. They had their patient's full and willing consent for the procedure and, as Dr Dubernard told a press conference at the time, 'My philosophy is very simple: we are doctors and we helped a patient with a very severe condition.' Another member of Isabelle's surgical team, Sylvie Testelin, added, 'It's easy to say we shouldn't have done it, but her life has changed; she goes shopping, she goes on holiday. Before she couldn't live. Before she didn't recognize herself, she scared herself. One can't live like this.'

The ethical issues surrounding the transplantation of human organs have also long been the subject of intense debate. From the outset it roused in some people fears of Dr Frankenstein-style tampering with the sanctity of human life. Culturally this was often difficult to accept, but it has become normalized in human medicine. When Christiaan Barnard transplanted the first human heart in the 1960s, the operation was celebrated in the media as an enormous breakthrough but there were also vociferous protests outside the hospital. Some sectors of society, especially the deeply religious ones, considered that this transplantation of the self, the soul, into a new body was sacrilege or even blasphemy. But it has become a far less emotive subject in the twenty-first century. Heart transplantation is now a routine practice that saves lives on a daily basis.

The transplantation of human facial tissues, however, continues to provoke ethical anxieties. But patients undergoing this form of reconstructive surgery around the world have regularly described the enormous transformation they have undergone in their lives after the transplantation of a new face, and it is important to realize, as pointed out by one of the surgeons who recently completed such a procedure, that these patients have actually in their lives had three different faces. They were born with a normal human face, they then sustained horrific damage to it and had to learn to cope with the altered version which was so abnormal that members of the public would stand, stare, point and even be horrified by the sight of it, and then an operation gave them a third, more normal-looking face. As a result, life began again for them.

A further ethical debate surrounds patients who, like Chrissy, have been blinded by facial trauma, leading critics to ask, in that event, for whose benefit the facial transplant has actually been carried out. They argue that blind people cannot see the reactions of those around them in public places or even in private, and thus are not exposed to the horrific feeling of being outcasts from human society. If that is the case, they say, why operate to give the blind person a new face when, quite apart from all the attendant risks of the procedure itself, the effects of immuno-suppressive drugs will also almost certainly shorten their lives?

Such arguments were called into question recently in the case of a young American man who underwent a face transplant despite having lost all vision in both eyes. After he had recovered from his operation, he described his small daughter sitting on his knee and the feeling of her kissing his new face – a sensation he had previously been unable to experience because his enormously scarred and damaged facial tissues were so numb he could not feel his daughter's touch. Even the slightest human contact is a necessary joy in our lives, and the man found the kiss from his daughter so incredibly life-affirming that it made him feel that all of his recent surgery and the life-long necessity for drugs to suppress his immune reaction were well worth every disadvantage they brought with them.

Of course, your face is inextricably bound up with your identity. An American nurse, Carmen Blandin Tarleton, had a face transplant in 2013 after an attack by her estranged husband, who doused her face with an industrial-strength detergent, left her with 80 per cent burns. Her doctors described it as 'the most horrific injury a human being could suffer', and by the time a suitable donor for a facial transplant had been found she had already endured fifty-eight separate bouts of surgery. After a further, seventeen-hour operation in 2013 she became the seventh person in the United States to receive a transplanted face. The recent spate of horrific attacks in the UK by people using acid to disfigure their victims suggests that the need for such transplants will only continue to grow.

At the time of her transplant, Carmen was not only suffering from the physical and psychological effects of disfigurement, caused both by her injuries and the surgery to ameliorate her symptoms, she also had to endure extreme levels of pain from the acid scars to her neck and the consequent restriction of her head and neck movement. Even to keep her head in an upright posture for any length of time was excruciating.

In a moving and inspiring interview with Kirsty Wark for the BBC's *Newsnight* programme in November 2015, Carmen said that when she decided to go ahead with a face transplant she was absolutely confident that this was the right treatment for her and had had no second thoughts whatsoever. 'When I decided that I was going to go forward and see if I was a candidate for a face transplant,' she said, 'I never looked back. I always had a certain confidence and security that that was what I needed at the time.'

That certainty was remarkable, given that as a nurse of twenty years' experience Carmen was only too well aware of the risks of rejection. She had undergone so much surgical intervention and had had blood transfusions from so many different donors that, despite the measures taken to deplete the immune-stimulating effect of transfused blood, she had developed antibodies to several of the markers that must be matched in order for tissues not to be rejected, even with powerful drugs suppressing the immune system.

With her team of doctors, she decided to take the chance and became the first person to have a transplant which was not a complete immune match for the donor facial tissue she would be receiving. She did so even though, despite the complexity of her surgery, there was no guarantee that she would be able to keep her new face. It was a horrific prospect, given that the scarred tissues had healed over her facial soft tissues and, should her new face be lost, it would leave her with an enormous defect and no way of helping it heal – in other words, she would have been left with an even more disfigured face, and this time incurably so.

'I knew that it was not a guarantee that I would be able to keep my new face,' Carmen said, 'but I always had a certain faith that it would work out.' Her faith appeared to be justified. As she said to Kirsty Wark, 'It's been almost three years now and it's doing well.'

The BBC interview also gave a remarkable insight into the effect on the human psyche of losing your face and then regaining a different one – and such operations are not a transformation of the original face to an entirely new one, but a transition from the horrifically damaged, scarred and extremely painful facial structure that has already replaced the face they were born with to something that, if not their original face, is at least recognizably human. Carmen felt that the fact that this treatment had been available to her, coupled with the reduction in her pain and need for powerful anti-necrotic drugs, had 'transformed my life much, much for the better and I am truly blessed'.

And when Kirsty Wark asked her about the concept of human identity, Carmen replied that she had never contemplated her own identity prior to the horrific injuries she suffered and the surgical journey that led to her face transplant. But then she added, 'Now that I have had the experience of being a disfigured person, and now a person that has a new face, it has been quite strange to look in the mirror nowadays, but I actually had my first dream last week of me with my new face. So we are very connected to our identity through our face. I have always concentrated on the core of who I am because my looks have changed so dramatically over a short period of time.'

At the time of her ground-breaking new procedure, good fortune was on the side of both Isabelle Dinoire and the treating team, because the dead patient who became the unwitting donor of facial tissues matched Isabelle for immune typing in all but one of the major categories that are tested prior to considering whether tissue can be tolerated by the recipient patient. The human immune system operates by recognition of self-tissue and rejection of any non-self-tissue. Any tissue not recognized as self-tissue by the immune cells (lymphocytes) on the surface of cells is attacked by the host's immune system. The only way to prevent this natural rejection of a transplanted organ or tissue is to mute the protective effect of the human immune system, but doing so exposes patients to an increased risk from other diseases, especially infections and, over time, cancers.

A phenomenon that has been noticed for some years in patients on immuno-suppressive therapy is that the normal tissues age at an accelerated rate because of the effect of certain of these drugs. This became evident in Isabelle's case as her transplanted face began to appear far more youthful than the rest of her facial soft tissues. She was undergoing what might simply have been the normal ageing process with a sagging of the facial structures and a loss of volume from the upper part of her face, except that this appeared to be accelerating in her early and mid-forties as a consequence of the immune suppression required to prevent the rejection of her new face.

Although the procedure had allowed Isabelle to enjoy, if not a normal life, at least more of a normal life than would have been possible had her terrible facial scarring been left untreated, her story had a tragic ending. Over the course of the ten years following her transplant, no doubt hastened by the immuno-suppressive drugs she was taking, she developed two cancers. She was ill for some time, and in April 2016 she finally lost her brave battle when her depleted immune system was no longer able to control the new growths of tumours in her body.

As yet, no full-face transplants have been carried out in the UK. The Glasgow unit where I now work, at the Queen Elizabeth University Hospital, was on the cusp of being the UK centre for facial transplants at one time, led by my colleague Colin MacIver. As is often the case, potential costs have been a barrier to our health board setting up the subsidiary facilities that would be needed (though most are on site anyway in the biggest hospital in Europe). But we have all the technical expertise – the immunology and the surgical skills – so when we have a suitable patient and the right donor we will carry out a full-face transplant.

It has been known for many decades that, following successful immune suppression for transplantation of organs such as the kidneys or the liver, patients are prone to developing tumours. My own surgical team has regularly treated patients with facial skin cancers that have developed following years of immune suppression after a kidney transplant. That was clear evidence, of course, of the effectiveness of the unsuppressed immune system in removing invading tumour cells and eradicating them before they got a grip on the tissues that could ultimately kill the patient. This led to the conclusion that the immune system could perhaps be harnessed and targeted at any human tumour in order to eradicate cancer cells, while leaving the host tissue intact.

One of the greatest challenges has been to establish why cancer cells do not trigger a strong immune response. It is clear that they have evolved a number of strategies to avoid detection by the body's natural defences, but research is now beginning to show us ways in which those strategies can be defeated, and without doubt immune therapies will play an increasingly prominent role in cancer treatment, especially in the head and neck cancers that I treat.

I'm closely involved in two clinical trials at my centre that may allow us to use the body's own immune responses to fight head and neck cancer more effectively. One, funded by Cancer Research UK (CRUK) and managed by the CRUK Centre for Drug Development, involves a drug, AMG 319, that has the potential to combat auto-immune conditions such as rheumatoid arthritis, but also inhibits cell proliferation, which has obvious implications for cancer treatment.

AMG 319 is designed to increase the ability of the body's white blood cells to identify tumours as alien to the body and then, just as they would with an infection, attack and destroy the cancer. There is still a long way to go before the clinical trial is complete but this kind of immune therapy offers the prospect of eliminating or at least shrinking tumours, which will make surgery and radiotherapy more effective and less debilitating for the patient, retain more of the patient's own healthy tissue, and reduce the risk of a recurrence of the cancer.

The other trial I'm involved in is called 'INSPIRE', run by IRX Therapeutics, and once more it is aiming to promote a coordinated, focused immune response by the body against cancerous cells. IRX is experimenting with incubating donor white cells in vitro in a fluid containing the molecules that white cells use to activate. When these white cells have multiplied in the fluid, they in turn produce chemokines (chemicals that further activate immune cells). When these are injected near the tumour in the patient's neck, there appears to be a boost to their own immune response: CD8 lymphocytes, cells that kill 'bad' cells, can then see and destroy cancer cells.

We are born with inherited immunities to some things, but others we develop in response to our environment, just as an inoculation of a very mild dose of a disease allows us to develop immunity to the full-strength disease. These adaptive immunities are obviously the ones we're interested in for cancer treatments. If we can find ways to develop and encourage them, the body will have not only its natural defences against viruses and other infections, but also an enhanced ability to detect cancer cells and neutralize them.

In early work before the INSPIRE trial was developed and opened, a patient's tumour reduced significantly, both in size and in cell activity, without any other treatment. If those results are confirmed by subsequent trials, it offers the prospect that some people will be able to avoid major surgery altogether, and some will have a shrinkage of their tumour so that their surgery is less morbid, less involved, less lengthy and less complicated.

I now chair a Phase 1 committee at Glasgow, purely to assess safety and approve or reject clinical trials of treatments at the very earliest stage of investigation. But as hard as we and other researchers try to make the process as safe as possible, clinical trials can never be entirely risk-free. The three-stage process is well under way. Phase 1 – how toxic is it and how is it handled by the body, and even do people die the moment you inject it? – has been successfully completed. The current trial is early Phase 2, studying fifty patients in the UK. Depending on outcomes, further trials such as a later Phase 2 to study larger numbers (maybe 200 patients nationally) may follow. Once that is complete, drugs will often roll on to Phase 3: a major study with hundreds more patients involved, to prove their effectiveness definitively. After that, if all has gone well, the next step is to seek the approval of the Food and Drug Administration in the United States and the MHRA (Medicines and Healthcare products Regulatory Agency) in the UK. We would then be able to start using those immune therapies to treat our head and neck cancer patients. So those therapies are not yet ready for clinical use and will not be ready this year or the next, but the time-frame for them to be available to patients worldwide should not be longer than just a few more short years.

We have already come a long way in cancer treatment, and continuing developments in chemotherapy, radiotherapy and immune therapy offer the prospect of even greater improvements. But while immune therapy gives us great hope for the future, it would be naive to imagine that the disease can ever be completely conquered. In any foreseeable future, curing cancer will never be possible for every patient. Still, the aim of cancer treatment is not confined to providing a cure. Extending life expectancy, palliating symptoms and improving patients' quality of life and functional status – measured either as survival time or, perhaps more usefully, disease-free survival time – remain hugely worthwhile aims.

16

ONE OF THE issues in my career I frequently reflect on is that, while I have been able to cure many hundreds of patients over the years and ease the pain and suffering of those I have been unable to help, none of this has eased the pain of the person whose illness first convinced me to become a surgeon – my own mother.

As a result of the polio that struck when she was very young, my mum's right foot dropped because of the loss of power to the muscle in her leg, which then shrank remarkably. There's not very much muscle at all below her knee, and that produces the aching pain that she has always suffered from. In the years before the post-polio pain syndrome was recognized, every time my mum went to see someone about the pain she was feeling, the orthopaedic team would assume it was caused by arthritis in her hip, just because that was a common complaint. However, the X-ray films they then took showed that there wasn't the degeneration of the joints that you would expect to see, so that forced them to think again.

It must have been so frustrating for her, because she knew she had all this discomfort and these aches and pains, but every time she sought medical help they would do an X-ray and say, 'Oh, it's not as bad as we thought.' Even worse, that carried with it the implicit assumption that she was making up her symptoms, or at the least exaggerating them.

So it was almost a vindication for her, decades later, when the post-polio pain syndrome was finally recognized. It showed absolutely clearly that polio viruses attack certain tissues; they attach to surface receptors which react differently on different types of tissues. The polio virus attacks the alpha motor neurone in the spinal cord, which is why it damages the motor innervation – the means by which nerve impulses are carried to the muscles. In a lot of undergraduate medical textbooks there's a full stop after that, and that's it: that's what polio does. But it's quite clear that it affects other parts of the nervous system as well, and that's what sets up the pain my mum has had to endure for over sixty years. In all that time I don't think she has ever been completely free of it.

This chronic, nagging pain meant that we could never go on a walk anywhere with her. Whenever we went on a trip to London for a few days, for example, even getting her up and down on the Tube or up the steps of a museum was a big issue. She couldn't walk very far at all, so in the end we had to stop doing it. Quite often we would see that she was making a big effort, like at the graduation ceremonies after my sister and I completed our degrees, and she'd be hoofing along and going for it, trying to ignore the pain, but we knew she'd pay the price for that over the next couple of days ... as would my dad, actually, because he'd get it in the neck! Latterly – I'd say for the last twenty-five years or so – whenever my parents have travelled they have always had to organize a wheelchair for her, and she's had to use it because of the pain that has resulted from her impaired mobility.

Despite this she has certainly always been highly motivated to get on and make things happen, and she's not been short of a hard word at times as well. But it must have been doubly difficult for her because as a woman, and as someone who was only four feet eleven inches tall and walked with a limp, I think she was quite often going in for medical appointments with her metaphorical fists already up, expecting to have to fight just so she wouldn't be taken for granted, ignored or patronized by the doctors she saw.

My mum has had all sorts of different drugs and treatments over the years – the sort of things that pain clinics would routinely run through, like tricyclics, which were originally designed as anti-depressants thirty years ago but have multiple effects and are quite good for phantom limb pain. Soldiers sometimes come back from Iraq or Afghanistan with limbs missing but still feeling severe pain, and when you ask 'Where is it?' they'll say, 'It's in the foot that's missing', because that's what it feels like. I've successfully prescribed tricyclics on many occasions for pain, but sadly in my mum's case they just didn't agree with her, so they were of no help to her.

When conventional medicine wasn't finding a solution, she even went to see a homeopath. Those sorts of alternative therapies tend to attract folk who, if not exactly in the 'last-chance saloon', are desperately looking for a remedy when they've pretty much exhausted the possibilities of regular medicine. But homeopathy proved to be of no use to her either.

Polio varies enormously in its effects, depending on which part of the motor nervous system it affects. Some polio patients couldn't breathe without respirators and they didn't live very long at all, others with less dramatic symptoms also died much younger than would normally be expected. My mum has lived to a good age, but the disease and its effects have continued throughout her life, and all our lives.

My dad has also been ill recently and undergoing radiotherapy, but at first he was reluctant to have the treatment. Part of the reason might be because in Scotland it is often incorrectly referred to as 'radium therapy', and there are pejorative associations with the word 'radium'. There was far less regulation of medical treatments in the early twentieth century and, following the discovery of radium and overblown claims about its curative properties, medical companies and salesmen rushed to produce patent medicines and quack cures containing it. It was added to toothpaste and even dissolved in bottled drinking water under the brand name Revigator. In the late 1940s, when workers who painted clock faces and watches with radium to make them glow in the dark were shown to be suffering from the effects of radium ingestion, and it was discovered that physical tolerance was much lower than expected and exposure to it caused long-term cell damage, the use of radium was dramatically curtailed. Despite this, some parts of the population in Scotland continue to insist on calling radiotherapy 'radium therapy' or 'having the radium', fuelling an illogical fear of it.

However, my dad is an engineer by background and knows a lot about cars, so I finally said to him, 'Listen, Dad, if you took the car to your garage and they told you some nonsense about it needing major repairs, you'd question it, challenge it, get the relevant information and then make your own decision about whether to go ahead, wouldn't you? So do me a favour and do the same with your healthcare. Don't be swayed by some old wives' tale about radium. Do the research, become as well informed as you can, and then act on that. And, Dad? Use the right terminology too, because it's not radium therapy, it's radiotherapy.' So he did that, and having done so, to my great relief, he decided to go ahead with the treatment, and is recovering well from it.

I began my surgical career by dividing my time between surgery and research, and they remain equal passions for me. Doing the surgery well and running a team efficiently is a hugely rewarding pursuit but, although it might be slightly trite to say it, if you're running a research project effectively and you get a successful answer from it, you can change things for tens of thousands of patients, not just the one you're operating on. Clinical research also raises the game in another way since it keeps the grey matter turning over. It's never routine and you're always looking to find new ways to improve your own practice and outcomes for your patients.

From the patients' point of view there are also benefits from their medical and surgical teams being involved in clinical trials because it's long been noted that if you're in such a trial, your results are better, irrespective of whether you're receiving the trial drug or just a placebo. It seems that it's not necessarily that the patients are in the clinical trial per se that makes the difference, but the fact that they are being treated by the people in that line of work, because the units carrying out research work operate to higher standards. There is also the 'Hawthorne effect', named after a man who carried out tests on the work patterns of factory workers. He established that people tend to feel better about their situation when it comes to things like clinical trials, not because anything has actually changed but simply because they know they're being studied.

In the head and neck cancer field, if you're treated at a unit that has a higher level of recruitment to clinical trials, then survival curves – not dying, in other words – are much better than in units that don't recruit many patients to trials,* and that's without even considering the results of units that don't recruit any patients to trials at all. If not quite running on empty, the NHS is always pretty close to the limit, so adding the extra capacity to the treatment side because there's a research team involved in a trial is also probably one of the reasons why patient outcomes are better. So there's a clear advantage, and you can see that in even the most basic ways. For example, there are extra people in a team if there is a trial running, so appointments are much less likely to be missed, scans get done on time, and so on.

The necessarily slow pace of clinical trials, with each phase subject to intensive scrutiny and analysis before we move on to the next, can be frustrating, particularly when nothing seems to have happened for six months or even a couple of years, but after, say, five years it's often remarkable how much things have progressed and improved. We're now in the middle of a culture change in our speciality, where research and development of new knowledge has become a core part of everyone's work. You do still get a few people rolling their eyes at that and saying, 'Can we not just get on with the job?' But the only answer to that is, 'Should we *never* improve, then? Should we not have moved on from using ether and chloroform?'

After being involved in research at the Beatson Laboratories while I was a registrar, I'm now back, full circle, working with

---

* Wuthrick et al, 'Institutional Clinical Trial Accrual Volume and Survival of Patients with Head and Neck Cancer', *Journal of Clinical Oncology*, Vol. 33 (January 2015), No. 2, pp.156-64.

Emma Shanks, a group leader at the Beatson who has actually had head and neck cancer herself. We're collaborating on a project analysing why some pre-cancer patches turn to cancer, measuring which bits are the highest risk and trying to identify them with a surface gel that we're also developing.

On the face of it the problem should not be so hard to solve because, after the skin, the second easiest site to examine on the body is inside the mouth. Patients are referred to us if they've got an odd-looking, usually red or white patch in their mouth. When a piece is biopsied under local anaesthetic, the pathology team will find some abnormal cells and then we have to decide what to do about that. If the patients smoke, we ask them to stop; if they drink a lot, we ask them to stop that too. However, some don't smoke or drink yet still have abnormal cells. The chances of the patch turning into cancer are unknown, but if it does, the consequences for the patient are often fatal. If we go ahead and try to remove it, we may leave some cells behind that may become cancerous or we may damage the function of the patient's mouth so that their quality of life is made worse without any certainty that the patch would ever have turned into cancer.

So the search for biomarkers to predict whether such patches will or will not become cancerous has been going on in the labs for years. Some progress has been made, but there are still many difficulties to overcome. How, for instance, do we know that we've biopsied the worst bit, and how can we tell where it starts and stops?

What are called tri-iodate studies may finally allow us to identify the pre-cancer cells since they don't have any glycogen (a substance deposited in bodily tissues as a store of carbohydrate) in them – a discovery that won German scientist Otto Warburg a Nobel Prize way back in 1931. It is now clear that if all the glycogen in a cell has been used up, it is an important sign that it's going to become a cancer cell very soon. We can exploit that on the surfaces of the mouth by painting on a tri-iodate solution, under which normal cells are a chocolate-brown colour but bad cells show as a pale yellow colour, so at last we may have a tool to show where the bad part starts and stops. We are examining how effective this is now in the LISTER trial, funded by the Oracle Cancer Trust and London Northwest Teaching Hospitals.

We still have a long way to go because at the moment the liquid we use to try to identify the pre-cancerous cells is a bit like metal polish: it not only tastes foul but it's toxic if you swallow too much of it, therefore we can only use it under general anaesthetic. So it's a bit of a Catch-22 situation: you only put someone on the operating list if you're going to remove the suspicious patch of mucosa, but you don't know if you need to do so, or indeed can do so, until you've used the stain.

We're currently trying to navigate a way around this dilemma by looking for a gel that does the same job but is not toxic and doesn't taste so bad. We could then use it in the outpatient clinic, do the biopsy and remove any pre-cancerous cells. That's what we're working on, and if we're successful, our working lives will be a lot less complicated, and some of our patients' lives will be considerably extended. So research is absolutely key.

As I reflect on my surgical career, I often hark back to the Harold Gillies era and think about how similar some things are today, but how very different other aspects are. To some extent what we do in Glasgow now to rebuild faces parallels what

Gillies and his colleagues started to do with the First World War wounded, but because of the continuing evolution of his techniques and the addition of laboratory services that were not available to him we're able to be much more precise in our surgery. For example, we provide a service for the dermatology team who perform Mohs micrographic surgery ('Mohs surgery' for short), named after Dr Frederic E. Mohs, who devised the technique for removing skin cancer lesions in 1938. It involves gradually removing layers of tissue and putting them under the microscope. The pathologists call back and tell the team to take a little more and we just keep going like that in stages until we're certain there's no more cancerous tissue left behind. It's a more accurate process, ensuring we take no more tissue than is absolutely necessary rather than estimating – which means pretty much guessing – how much to remove. The downside is that doing it in stages like that can mean we're left with a rather less 'reconstruction friendly' site for the transplanted flap than might otherwise be the case.

Surgical techniques are constantly evolving, sometimes in major leaps but more often in tiny, incremental phases, and apparently minuscule changes and adaptations can end up saving a life. Even major changes in medical practice can be subject to further refinements. For example, when I first did advanced trauma life support many years ago, using a tourniquet was regarded as a bad plan because if you tied it wrong, you obstructed the venous outflow but didn't block the arterial inflow, so you sprayed even more blood over a damaged limb and out of a damaged body. However, in the war in Iraq, and particularly when treating the casualties from IEDs in Iraq and Afghanistan, the use of tourniquets proved to be life-saving:

if you put rapid-pressure tourniquets on both legs, wounded soldiers didn't bleed to death.

A much smaller but by no means insignificant gain I've made in my own operating technique has been to reduce the pressure at which tourniquets are applied. A tourniquet used to be routinely set at 250 (on an arm) to 350 (on a leg) millimetres of mercury pressure (mmHg). Under anaesthetic, your systolic blood pressure is usually no more than about 110 mmHg, so you only need the tourniquet to be around 50 above that not to have any bleeding while operating. Keeping tourniquets to this lower pressure also means we get less crush injury of the blood vessels and fewer complications at the flap donor site as a result. I have my sister Janet to thank for that, because she discovered that turning the tourniquet down reduced ill effects following knee surgery, and when she told me about it, I tried it and then adopted it as part of my own surgical practice.

We have made hundreds of other refinements – some major, some minor – to the techniques that Harold Gillies pioneered almost exactly a hundred years ago, and we also now benefit from materials, drugs and techniques that were unknown back then. We try not to overuse antibiotics now, but thank God we've got them, because back in the days before they were discovered Gillies' patients were constantly at risk of an overwhelming, and fatal, infection. They knew about antisepsis (from Joseph Lister) and asepsis (from John MacEwan, both of Glasgow Royal Infirmary) by then, and they were using gloves and 'no touch' techniques, but anaesthesia wasn't as advanced, the drugs weren't as sophisticated, the conditions were dirtier, and the tubes they used for tracheostomies were made of rubber and lacked a cuff, whereas when we do a tracheostomy now we have all sorts of synthetic materials and inflatable cuffs available to us.

We have new painkilling drugs that have a much shorter half-life and fewer side-effects. We have anti-emetics, and can now much better control the vomiting that is an inevitable side-effect of the anaesthetic process (hence the 'nil by mouth' instruction prior to operations). We also have a better under-standing of the physiology of injury and operations, and I'm now working on a systematic review of enhancing recovery after major head and major neck surgery. Although it has been very much in vogue in other types of major operations, this has never been properly grasped to minimize complications such as infection and lung injury in our patients. Enhanced recovery means less impact from the operation and fewer complications, and a lot of the process is aimed at mitigating the human stress response to injury and the operation to cure it.

Ninety-five per cent of Harold Gillies' work during and after the First World War was in repairing battlefield injuries caused by shrapnel, bullets and explosions. Despite the rise in gun crime in the UK and the armed police response to it, I still don't treat that many gunshot and blast victims because wounded soldiers today are treated by the expert (and, after a quarter of a century of near continuous military actions and terrorist outrages, very experienced) specialist maxillofacial trauma teams at the Royal Centre for Defence Medicine at the Queen Elizabeth Hospital, Birmingham. But although civilian shootings are still relatively few and far between compared to the week-on-week mayhem in American cities, they do occur.

One recent, very sad case involved Barry, a soldier who had been due to go back to Afghanistan with his unit, but because of the injuries he had sustained on his previous tour of duty he was told he was unfit for further active service and would be medically discharged while his mates returned to the country without him. Barry insists that what followed had nothing to do with any depression resulting from that, nor from post-traumatic stress disorder from his earlier service in Afghanistan. 'The Army is not in any way to blame for what I did,' he told me.

Whatever the cause, Barry went down to his basement and tried to commit suicide with an antique shotgun he owned. He held the barrels against the underside of his chin, intending to fire it straight up through his head and into his brain. Had he achieved that he would have been killed instantly but, like many other attempted suicides by shotgun, as he leaned down to reach the trigger, without realizing it he tilted the angle of the barrels and his head, and when he pulled the trigger, instead of killing himself he blew off the front of his face. The impact of both barrels blasted right through his chin, his jawbone and his teeth, ripped through the soft tissues of his lips and lower face and tore off part of his nose as well.

Because his wounds had been sustained by his own hand rather than in combat when serving with his unit, Barry was not taken to the Royal Centre for Defence Medicine, but instead was treated at an NHS hospital. He underwent multiple oper-ations that painstakingly, and painfully, reconstructed the lost and damaged structures of his face, rebuilding his nose and replacing the teeth lost along with his blast-damaged jawbone. The end is now almost in sight: he needs only a couple more minor 'fine-tuning' operations to complete the restoration of his face to the appearance he had before that fateful day. Barry realizes only too well how fortunate he is to have been granted a second chance at life and is determined to embrace it and all its possibilities.

Barry recently spoke to me about this episode in his life, having gone through counselling after recovering from his injuries. 'I want to be very clear this had nothing to do with the military,' he said. 'I had reached a stage where I had had enough and just wanted to go. The most mortifying thing about it is that with all my specialist training and years of experience, I missed from point-blank range!'

He also told me about how it had felt to get his face back. 'Craig Wales [my consultant colleague in Glasgow] says different, but I know he really saved my life. He gave me back my face, and I can't thank him enough for that, but the positive attitude of him and the whole team absolutely saved me and gave me back the strength to move on in my life. I am so glad to have this further chance and further time. I couldn't do it without my face back.'

The crucial role of the human face as the proof of our identity is clear from Barry's words and may be even more pronounced today in the era of the 'selfie' – the modern equivalent of the historical portrait, but available to everyone with a smartphone.

One week in eight I focus on trauma injuries, dealing with facial trauma caused by anything from a kicking or a beating with a baseball bat to a road traffic accident, a fall from a great height or, very occasionally, a gunshot or something even more unexpected. I've treated hundreds of trauma victims over the years, but one of my more bizarre cases was Larry, a frail, elderly man with Parkinson's disease who, wanting to cut a cat-flap in his back door for his pet, had attempted to do so with an angle-grinder. It is not a tool you would want an inexperienced person to be using, least of all one with the tremors and general frailty associated with his condition, and the results were regrettably predictable. Wearing a helmet and protective visor, he stooped over the angle-grinder and began trying to make a cut in the bottom of the door. However, the tool kicked back, knocking off his helmet and slicing his face right down the middle, leaving a wound that was more analogous to a sabre cut than a ballistic trauma. The cut was so clean that all the facial bones and tissues were still there, just neatly parted down the middle. The operation to reconnect the two halves of his face proved to be one of the most successful I and Dave Sutton have ever performed and it took only three hours to fix it, using micro-surgery and large stents (surgical tubes) to stop his nasal cavity healing shut.

His daughter had seen him just after the accident when he appeared on her doorstep (she lived next door), and had greeted his lacerated and profusely bleeding arrival with the words 'Oh, what have you done now, Dad?', which suggested that Larry was no stranger to mishaps that might end in the Emergency Medicine department.

When he appeared in my consulting rooms a few weeks later it was almost impossible to detect that there had ever been anything wrong with him, but to my surprise he appeared to be a little downcast.

'What's the matter, Larry?' I said. 'Are you not happy with what we've done for you?'

'Oh no, doctor,' he replied, 'I'm very happy with that. It's my kids.'

'How so?'

'Well, they've taken my angle-grinder off me.'

His deadpan delivery meant that it took me a few moments to assess whether this was Parkinson's disease or humour, but my doubts were cleared up when Larry burst out laughing, together with Bev my clinic nurse, and finally me.

If he could come back to life today, Harold Gillies might be surprised at the uses to which angle-grinders can be put, but he would be staggered at some of the medical and surgical advances that have taken place since his time. And we are now entering a new surgical world that would have seemed like science fiction even to us only a few years ago. As well as increasingly complex facial transplants, plans to 'roboticize' some forms of surgery are well advanced, with new techniques in development or undergoing medical trials, and some already in use. The Da Vinci robotic system, where surgeons operate a computerized console and the actual surgery is carried out by the robot, is already in widespread use. If a patient is referred to us with a neck lump that signals a secondary cancer in a lymph node, for example, but with no indication of the site of the primary cancer, we can use the robot to access the base of the tongue and the tonsils without having to cut open the patient's face and take off the surface tissue to discover where the cancer has come from.

Other new robotic systems are under development, including the British-designed Versius, the world's smallest surgical robot, which uses low-cost technology originally designed for mobile phones and space industries to mimic the movements of the human wrist and hand more precisely than other robots. It can be used in a wide range of laporoscopic procedures, including ear, nose and throat surgery, and prostate, hernia and colorectal operations. The robot allows us to make a series of small incisions rather than the more large-scale, traditional open surgery, reducing patients' post-operative pain and surgical complications, and improving their speed of recovery.

Scientists in the Hamlyn Centre at Imperial College, London, are also trialling other advanced technologies that may soon be made available to surgeons. They include an 'iKnife' (Intelligent Knife), which instantly tests the smoke generated as it burns through tissue for signs of the molecules found in cancerous cells, offering the prospect of more precise excision of tumours, thus leaving more healthy tissue behind.

An optical biopsy probe is also being developed, so powerful that it will enable surgeons to identify cell structures linked to cancer that may be invisible under normal imaging, without the need to resort to the much more invasive collection of tissue samples needed for the traditional biopsy. Another idea in development aims to overlay previous X-rays, MRI scans and other imaging on to the patient's tissue to help guide the surgeon as he operates. A 'gaze-tracking' system, allowing a surgeon to direct robot instruments simply by moving his eyes, is also planned. 'We are entering a new age of precision surgery,' Professor Guang-Zhong Yang, the director of the Hamlyn Centre, told the *Sunday Times*. 'We want to enhance surgeons with robots that give them almost superhuman powers to image and diagnose damaged tissues, and the dexterity to repair them.'

New techniques and instruments are continually refining and improving maxillofacial surgery, but immune therapy and other 'magic bullet' therapies may one day transform cancer treatment by dramatically reducing or even eliminating the need for surgical excision of tumours. However, whatever happens in that field, there will always be a need for maxillofacial surgeons to repair and restore the looks of victims of facial trauma, whatever its cause. Nor is there any foreseeable end to the demand for purely cosmetic treatments. The ever-growing pressure on people, men and women alike, to have 'the right look' for our image-obsessed age is bound to lead to an increasing demand for surgical and other treatments to enhance what nature has given us, or counter the effects of ageing. In this era, probably more than any other, the way we look dictates how others regard us, and often how we regard ourselves.

Some people actively want to be noticed – to stand out in a crowd – but in the right way, as an object of interest or attraction, not one provoking pity or revulsion. I suspect that most people simply want to pass in a crowd without drawing unwanted attention to themselves. The ability to do that is something most of us take for granted, but those who are 'unusual looking' or physically disfigured may never be able to do so. A life lived behind an 'imperfect' face is a life diminished. The maxillofacial surgeon's role – and it is our pride and our joy as well – is to be able to correct those imperfections and allow the 'person behind the mask' to emerge and live their life to the full.

For all the changes that have already taken place in surgery and in society, and the interval of a hundred years that separates us, like Harold Gillies, I and my peers operate – in both senses of the word – in a continuum. Just as he did a century before us, my team not only rebuilds shattered faces but shattered lives as well.

The father of a patient I'd successfully treated once told me,

'I think it's amazing what you do.' I thanked him for the compliment, but said, 'Actually, what's really amazing is Harold Gillies and those who came after him, who first thought of the techniques we use and pioneered the transfer of tissue around the human body. He invented the techniques, tried them and got away with them, and that truly is astonishing, because if you started from scratch, knowing only what Harold Gillies knew at the start of the First World War, would you think it was OK to take a chunk of skin from someone's thigh, stick it over a hole in their face, and that it would somehow be all right?'

I have never lost the joy of seeing a damaged face restored after corrective surgery. Even surgically cleaning and closing a large laceration gives rise to a profound sense of relief that is undiminished after over twenty years in my speciality. Restoring those faces returns life to the owners, giving them back their self-esteem and the confidence to go back out into the world and face society without being greeted with looks of horror, or seeing people turn aside to avoid them. For people who might have just about given up hope of ever doing so, it offers the chance of normal human relationships, and the prospect of a return to a fulfilling life of gainful employment.

Harold Gillies did this for the many hundreds of soldiers he treated, and he also gifted to us new methods of saving the human face. Moreover, he did so at a time when the welfare state was no more than a pipe-dream and when a man with a disfigured appearance might never obtain a job.

Helping restore the human face still feels like one of the most powerful gifts a surgeon can bestow. Standing in the operating theatre, scrubbed, behind a face mask, in the bright light of the operating lamps, hands encased in surgical gloves and breathing the sharp tang of antiseptic, I often have cause to reflect on the gifts bestowed on us today by those terribly wounded soldiers and their pioneering facial surgeon Harold Delf Gillies.

There is no hiding place for maxillofacial surgeons. We have to be psychologists as well as surgeons, and our work is there for all to see, quite literally 'as plain as the nose on your face'. There are great successes, but there are also some heart-breaking failures, like Michelle and all the others buried in my 'cemetery of regrets'. Surgeons – and, even more so, our patients – have to face the consequences of that.

As I write these final words, I am on call in Glasgow. This weekend I have cared for a ward full of surgically treated and facially reconstructed cancer patients and, with the rest of the maxillofacial team, assessed and treated many other patients presenting with damaged faces. A professional athlete, injured while playing elite rugby, had facial bones reduced together and plated with precision titanium plates and screws. Two children bitten on the face by family dogs had ripped wounds surgically cleaned, revised and closed. Three men with facial cuts and fractures after bar fights and a number of patients with severe infections, most arising from bad teeth, had surgery, one helicoptered in from the North of Scotland urgently so that the swelling from it did not crush his windpipe, preventing him from breathing. We have operated to restore the faces and identities of these people over the last two days using medical, dental and advanced twenty-first-century surgical expertise acquired over three decades of training. They are all getting better and some have gone home already.

Today, arriving at the ward at eight a.m. on a cold Sunday morning, I found a present left for me in the doctors' room. It was from Tony, a lovely, larger-than-life quantity surveyor who underwent major surgery for a rare sarcoma cancer in his face two years ago. With the parcel there was a card, and in it he had written, 'Thank you for saving my life and my looks, and for being a friend when I needed one most.'

I think mine is the most rewarding job in the world.

Acknowledgements

I am grateful to the many gifted people who taught and trained me at various stages of my life and career. I was very lucky to train with a group of maxillofacial surgeons who remain my best friends. My thanks also go to all the dedicated and skilful surgical, medical and nursing staff with whom I've worked over the years.

I am particularly indebted to all of the patients who have been under my care and from whom I have learned, especially those who have allowed me to write about their journey, and in some cases their destination.

I write scientific articles regularly, but telling the story of those patients and my speciality required a different skill-set and I'm very grateful to Mark Lucas at Lucas Alexander Whitley for his insight and enthusiasm, and to Doug Young and his team at Penguin Random House for their skill and professionalism.

Special thanks to Drew Hanson for additional research, emotional intelligence and calmness under stress.

Finally, and most importantly, thank you to Lorna, James and Katherine who, realizing that I work best under pressure, have given me decades of patience and love.

Index

INDEX

About the Author

Jim McCaul graduated with honours in both Medicine and Dentistry from the University of Glasgow. He completed his undergraduate studies in 1997, winning ten prizes and medals, then completed basic surgical training, gaining the FRCS Diploma in 1999, and entered higher training in the West of Scotland, London and Florida.

In 2005 he completed a PhD in Molecular Oncology (Telomere Function and Radio Sensitivity) at the Cancer Research UK (CRUK) Beatson Laboratories in Glasgow, and won the West of Scotland Head and Neck Prize, the Scottish OMFS Society Prize three times, and the European Head and Neck Golden Award during training. He was appointed Consultant Surgeon at the Bradford Teaching Hospitals in West Yorkshire in 2006 and worked there for eight years, developing clinical research into head and neck cancers that resulted in a team of seven research staff and over 850 patients being recruited to clinical studies.

He became Consultant Maxillofacial/Head and Neck Surgeon at the Royal Marsden Hospital, London, and Northwick Park Hospital, London, in April 2014. He was later the Director of Research and Development at Northwick Park. To his eleven national and international awards he added the British Association of Oral and Maxillofacial Surgeons (BAOMS) President's Award for research optimizing patient care in major surgery in 2012, and the BAOMS Surgery Prize in 2014, in recognition of his international reputation and contribution in the head and neck field. His team also won the BAOMS Norman Rowe Clinical Research Prize in 2014.

In 2017 he was appointed Consultant Surgeon in Maxillofacial/

Head and Neck Surgery at the Queen Elizabeth University Hospital, Glasgow, returning to the highest incidence site for facial and head and neck cancer in the UK. He is currently the National Research Lead for Maxillofacial/Head and Neck Research in the UK, and Research Lead for BAOMS. He is Chief Investigator of the CRUK LIHNCS trial, which successfully recruited 419 patients to time and target – an international first for a mouth cancer surgical clinical trial. He has been and is Principal Investigator for twenty other trials. His research interests lie in the early detection of face and mouth cancers and minimizing impact and optimizing outcomes from head and neck cancer treatment. He also researches in effectively treating and curing after-effects of treatment such as osteoradionecrosis (ORN). He is co-investigator in a further eight clinical trials in the UK and collaborates with colleagues in Europe and North America. These include analysis of new technologies for free flap monitoring and new pharmacological treatments for ORN and immunotherapy for cancer treatment.

He was associate editor of the *British Journal of Oral and Maxillofacial Surgery* for three years until 2014, is on the editorial board of the journal, and reviews for twelve other international medical research journals. He is assistant editor of the *International Journal of Surgery* and the author of five book chapters and fifty-seven scientific papers. In addition he has presented and published more than 130 research abstracts at national and international meetings. He sits on the Council and Endowments Committee of BAOMS, is a council member of the British Association of Head and Neck Oncologists and is a board member for the ethical tissue collection board at the Institute for Cancer Therapeutics, University of Bradford. He is currently Lead Clinician for Head and Neck Cancer in his native West of Scotland and Chair of the Phase 1 Committee for the NHS Greater Glasgow and Clyde, evaluating all 'first in human' studies.